INTERMITTENT FASTING FOR WOMEN OVER 50

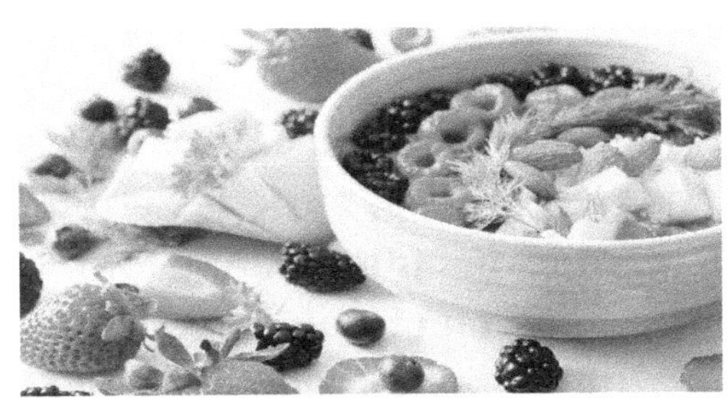

A Comprehensive Guide to Boost Energy, Lose Stubborn Weight and Improve Hormonal Health

LYNNE Q. CHAPMAN

TABLE OF CONTENTS

INTRODUCTION   **9**

Overview of Intermittent Fasting   11

How Does Intermittent Fasting Benefit Women in Their 50's?   12

Considerations for Age-Related Changes   14

What Happens to Your Body When You Fast?   16

Different Methods of Intermittent Fasting   19

The Science Behind Intermittent Fasting   21

CHAPTER ONE   **25**

CUSTOMISING INTERMITTENT FASTING FOR WOMEN OVER 50   25

Hormonal Changes and Menopause   25

Addressing hormonal imbalances   26

Essential nutrients for women over 50.   28

Adequate caloric intake   30

Micronutrient considerations   31

CHAPTER TWO   **35**

GETTING STARTED WITH INTERMITTENT FASTING   35

A. Preparing Mentally and Physically   35

B. Creating a Fasting Schedule   36

Finding the Fasting Pattern That's Perfect for You   36

Gradual Transition into Intermittent Fasting   38

Frequently Asked Questions   39

Addressing Misconceptions   41

CHAPTER THREE   **43**

NUTRIENT-DENSE FOODS FOR WOMEN
OVER 50   43

Key Nutrient-Dense and Fast Friendly
Foods/drinks: 43

Meal Planning Tips   45

Tips for a Successful Intermittent Fasting 46

CHAPTER FOUR   **47**

NUTRIENT-DENSE BREAKFAST OPTIONS 47

Protein-Packed Quinoa Breakfast Bowl   47

Chia Seed Pudding   48

Green Smoothie   49

Flaxseed and Berry Breakfast Parfait   50

Cinnamon-Spiced Baked Apple Oatmeal   52

Quinoa Power Bowl   53

Salmon Avocado Toast   54

Turmeric Golden Oatmeal   55

Sweet Potato and Spinach Frittata   57

Salmon and Avocado Breakfast Wrap   58

Greek Yogurt Parfait with Granola and
Berries   59

Almond Butter and Banana Overnight
Oats   60

Turmeric and Ginger Smoothie   61

Egg and Veggie Breakfast Skillet   62

Cauliflower and Kale Breakfast Hash   64

Mango and Coconut Chia Pudding   65

Blueberry and Almond Smoothie Bowl   66

Coconut Flour Pancakes with Mixed

Berries 67

Spinach and Feta Omelette 68

Cauliflower and Spinach Breakfast Burrito 70

CHAPTER SIX 73

SALAD RECIPES 73

Superfood Kale and Quinoa Salad 73

Nutty Spinach and Berry Salad 74

Cabbage and Edamame Slaw 76

Mediterranean Chickpea Salad 77

Quinoa and Black Bean Fiesta Salad 78

Vibrant Veggie Delight Salad 80

Quinoa & Chickpea Power Salad 81

Citrus Bliss Shrimp Salad 82

Mango Tango Quinoa Salad 83

Broccoli Almond Crunch Salad 84

CHAPTER SEVEN 87

VEGETABLE RECIPES 87

Broccoli and Cauliflower Salad 87

Sweet Potato and Black Bean Chili 88

Zucchini Noodles with Pesto 89

Balsamic Glazed Roasted Brussels Sprouts 90

Carrot Ginger Soup 90

Radiant Roasted Vegetable Medley 92

Savory Spinach Stuffed Mushrooms 93

Cauliflower & Turmeric Mash 94

Zesty Lemon Garlic Asparagus 95

Sweet Potato Kale Hash 96

CHAPTER EIGHT 99

FISH/SEA FOOD RECIPES 99

 Grilled Salmon Fillet with Asparagus 99

 Tequila Lime Shrimp Zoodles 100

 Harissa Fish with Bulgur Salad 101

 Mediterranean Fish Gratin 103

 Succulent Lemon Herb Salmon 104

 Zesty Shrimp and Avocado Salad 105

 Miso Glazed Cod with Sesame Broccoli 106

 Spicy Garlic Butter Lobster Tails 108

 Coconut Lime Cilantro Grilled Fish Tacos 109

CHAPTER NINE **111**

POULTRY RECIPES 111

 Turmeric Infused Grilled Chicken 111

 Lemon Rosemary Baked Turkey Thighs 112

 Mango Chili Lime Chicken Skewers 113

 Spinach and Feta Stuffed Chicken Breast 115

 Crispy Garlic Parmesan Chicken Tenders 116

 Balsamic Glazed Rosemary Chicken 117

 Sesame Ginger Glazed Chicken Stir-Fry 118

 Pomegranate Glazed Chicken Salad 120

 Mediterranean Chicken Skillet 121

 Cajun Spiced Chicken Lettuce Wraps 123

CHAPTER TEN **125**

MEAT RECIPES 125

 Ginger Garlic Glazed Beef Stir-Fry 125

 Lemon Herb Turkey Skillet 127

 Cumin Spiced Lamb Kebabs 128

Mushroom and Spinach Stuffed Pork Tenderloin 131

Orange Glazed Teriyaki Chicken 132

Sesame Ginger Glazed Salmon 134

Tomato Basil Turkey Meatballs 135

Bacon-Wrapped Asparagus Stuffed Chicken 137

Citrus-Infused Grilled Chicken 138

Sesame Ginger Turkey Meatballs 139

Mediterranean Lamb Skewers 141

Chili Lime Beef Stir-Fry 142

Coconut Lime Chicken Curry 143

CHAPTER ELEVEN 145

SNACK RECIPES 145

Dark Chocolate Avocado Mousse 145

Turmeric Almond Energy Bites 146

Greek Yogurt Berry Parfait 147

Chickpea and Roasted Red Pepper Hummus 148

Walnut and Date Protein Bars 150

Edamame and Avocado Dip 151

Cucumber and Salmon Roll-Ups 152

Black bean and Quinoa Stuffed Bell Peppers 153

Kale and Sweet Potato Chips 155

Protein-Packed Cottage Cheese with Berries 156

CHAPTER TWELVE 159

DESSERTS RECIPES 159

Cocoa-Dusted Almond Butter Banana Bites 159

Pomegranate and Greek Yogurt Parfait 160

Almond Flour Blueberry Muffins 161

Coconut and Matcha Green Tea Energy Bites 162

Turmeric Golden Milk Popsicles 164

Protein-Packed Greek Yogurt Parfait 165

Sweet Potato and Cinnamon Muffins 166

Mango and Coconut Chia Popsicles 167

Baked Apple with Cinnamon and Walnuts 168

CHAPTER THIRTEEN 171

BEVERAGES, HERBAL TEAS AND SMOOTHIES 171

Mango Tango Smoothie 171

Green Goddess Detox Smoothie 173

Turmeric Spice Golden Milk 175

Coconut Berry Hydration Elixir 176

Pineapple Ginger Zing Smoothie 177

Beetroot Berry Power Smoothie 178

Cinnamon Apple Pie Smoothie 179

Matcha Mint Refresher 180

Orange Creamsicle Smoothie 181

Cranberry Citrus Antioxidant Infusion 183

Blueberry Basil Brain Boost Smoothie 184

Peaches and Cream Protein Smoothie 185

Minty Watermelon Quencher 186

APPENDIX 189

Your Daily Planner 189

CONCLUSION 193

INTRODUCTION

The Intermittent Fasting Cookbook for Women Over 50 is a comprehensive guide that provides you with all the information you need to get started with intermittent fasting. As a woman over 50, you've likely noticed some changes in your body and health. Hormonal fluctuations, slowing metabolism, and other age-related factors can make it challenging to maintain an optimal health. But what if there was a way to turn back the clock, boost your metabolism, and improve your overall health and well-being?

Intermittent fasting, as revealed within the pages of this cookbook, transcends the realm of traditional diets. It's not about deprivation but rather about embracing a rhythmic approach to eating that aligns with the body's natural cycles.This simple practice involves cycling between periods of eating and fasting, allowing your body to reset and recharge. It has emerged as a powerful tool for women in their 50s and beyond.

But intermittent fasting is not just a weight loss tool, but has been shown to offer other numerous health benefits. Numerous studies show that fasting can improve your metabolism, mental health, and possibly prevent some cancers. It can also prevent certain muscle, nerve, and joint disorders which can affect women over 50. Intermittent fasting can also promote ketosis, which may help with hunger management and mental acuity, improve cardiovascular risk markers, potentially reverse type 2 diabetes, enhance the circadian rhythm, and activate a cellular longevity program called autophagy.

With practical advice and delicious recipes, this comprehensive resource will help you incorporate intermittent fasting into your lifestyle, promoting healthy aging, optimal health and well-being.

This cookbook delicately addresses the unique considerations of women in their 50s. Beyond the practical recipes, it delves into the science behind intermittent fasting, acknowledging the hormonal shifts and age-related changes. It offers not just meals but a roadmap—a culinary guide designed to navigate the nuanced landscape of menopause, hormonal imbalances, and the desire for lasting vitality. Thus, the cookbook provides age-specific fasting guidelines and tips for success.

It will become a reassuring companion, answering the innermost questions that echo in the minds of women embarking on this journey.

Overview of Intermittent Fasting

Intermittent fasting (IF) is not just a diet; it's a time-restricted eating pattern designed to optimize the body's natural cycles of digestion and repair. At its core, IF involves alternating periods of eating and fasting, creating windows of time where food intake is deliberately limited. The principle is simple but profound—it allows the body to tap into stored energy, promoting a range of physiological benefits.

Transitioning from a state of fed to fasting triggers metabolic shifts. During the fasting period, the body exhausts its immediate glycogen stores and begins utilizing fat for energy. This metabolic flexibility not only aids in weight management but also initiates a cascade of cellular repair processes, promoting longevity and overall well-being. There are several different methods of intermittent fasting, such as the 16/8 method (16 hours of fasting followed by an 8-hour eating window) and the 5:2 method (fasting for 5 days followed by 2 days of eating).

How Does Intermittent Fasting Benefit Women in Their 50's?

Intermittent fasting has been shown to have various health benefits for women over 50, including:

- **Weight loss**: Intermittent fasting can lead to weight loss by promoting ketosis (which may help with hunger management and mental acuity) and reducing calorie intake during eating windows.

- **Improved insulin sensitivity**: Fasting has been shown to improve insulin sensitivity, which can be beneficial for individuals with diabetes or prediabetes, women with PCOS, and other metabolic disorders.

- **Cardiovascular health:** Intermittent fasting has been associated with improved cardiovascular risk markers, such as reduced blood pressure and cholesterol levels.

-**Increased Longevity and Disease Prevention:** Some studies suggest that fasting has been linked to increased lifespan and reduced risk of age-related diseases.

It may also help prevent certain cancers, muscle disorders, and promote overall healthy aging.

 - Enhancing the circadian rhythm (24-hour wake-sleep cycle)

- Activating a cellular longevity program called autophagy

-Improved gut health: Fasting can help promote a healthy gut microbiome, which is crucial for overall health.

-Reduced stress and improved mood: Intermittent fasting can help regulate cortisol levels, reducing stress and improving mood.

-Easier weight management: Intermittent fasting can help boost metabolism, making it easier to maintain a healthy weight.
- **Enhanced cognitive function:** Fasting has been shown to increase levels of BDNF, a protein that promotes neural growth and protects against cognitive decline.

-Reduced inflammation: Intermittent fasting can reduce inflammation, which is associated with numerous chronic diseases.

Furthermore, IF has been shown to support cognitive function, a key concern for women over 50. The reduction in oxidative stress during fasting periods contributes to enhanced brain health, promoting mental clarity and resilience. Additionally, IF has been linked to hormonal balance, addressing changes associated with menopause and promoting overall hormonal well-being.

It is essential to consult with a healthcare professional before starting intermittent fasting, especially for those with certain medical conditions or nutritional needs. Keep in mind that individual experiences may vary, and it is crucial to listen to your body and adjust your fasting practices accordingly.

Considerations for Age-Related Changes

As women age, our metabolism and nutritional needs change. Biological shifts such as decreased muscle mass and alterations in hormone levels become more pronounced. Intermittent fasting, when tailored to these considerations, can be a powerful tool. Maintaining adequate protein intake during eating windows becomes crucial to preserve lean muscle mass, addressing the natural decline that occurs with age.

Moreover, IF can be adapted to accommodate fluctuations in energy levels and potential nutrient deficiencies associated with aging. It is essential to incorporate a nutrient-dense diet during eating windows, emphasizing foods rich in vitamins, minerals, and antioxidants to support overall health.

So, women over 50 may need to adjust their fasting windows and dietary choices to ensure they are meeting their age-specific needs. Some age-related changes that may affect intermittent fasting include:

- Hormonal changes, such as menopause, which can promote increased abdominal fat, osteoporosis, and accelerated muscle loss
- Slowed metabolism, which can lead to stubborn body fat

- Musculoskeletal health, as fasting has been shown to promote hormone secretion from the thyroid, which can promote bone health and help prevent bone fractures

In conclusion, intermittent fasting transcends the confines of a conventional diet—it's a lifestyle approach that aligns with the natural rhythms of the body. For women over 50, the benefits extend beyond weight management, offering a pathway to enhanced metabolic health, cognitive function, and hormonal balance. By understanding the principles and customizing the approach to age-related changes, intermittent fasting becomes a valuable tool in promoting a vibrant and resilient life.

What Happens to Your Body When You Fast?

Fasting is not just a period of abstaining from food; it's a physiological and psychological journey that unfolds within the intricate workings of your body. As you embark on a fast, typically initiated after several hours of not eating, your body undergoes an initial phase of adjustment. Glycogen, stored in the liver and muscles, serves as the primary energy source during the early hours of a fast. Once glycogen reserves are depleted, the body transitions into a state of ketosis—a metabolic state where it starts utilizing stored fat for energy. Let's delve into the profound changes that occur during a fast, shedding light on the intricate processes that contribute to both short-term and long-term health benefits.These changes can be broadly categorized into the following aspects:

Physical Changes

- **Increased fat oxidation:** During fasting, your body burns fat for energy instead of carbohydrates, leading to increased fat oxidation.

- **Ketosis**: Fasting triggers a process called ketosis, where the body breaks down fat into ketones for energy. This can help with hunger management and mental acuity.

- **Cellular Repair and Autophagy:** One of the most remarkable aspects of fasting is its role in promoting autophagy—a cellular recycling process. During a fast, cells break down and remove damaged components, fostering renewal and optimizing cellular function. This process has been associated with longevity and a reduced risk of various age-related diseases.

- **Reduced inflammation:** Intermittent fasting has been associated with reduced inflammation, which may contribute to its health benefits.

- **Hormonal Regulation:** Fasting triggers a delicate dance of hormones that play a pivotal role in metabolic regulation. Insulin levels drop, signaling the body to switch from a storage to a burning mode. Simultaneously, human growth hormone (HGH) increases, facilitating fat breakdown and muscle preservation. This hormonal symphony not only supports weight loss but also contributes to cellular repair and regeneration.

- **Blood Sugar Regulation:** Fasting has a profound impact on blood sugar levels. As the body transitions into using stored energy, blood sugar levels stabilize. This is particularly beneficial for individuals with insulin resistance, as fasting helps improve insulin sensitivity, reducing the risk of type 2 diabetes.

Psychological Changes
- **Cognitive Benefits**: Beyond the physical realm, fasting influences cognitive function. The increase in brain-derived neurotrophic factor (BDNF) during fasting supports brain health, enhancing learning, memory, and overall cognitive performance. Fasting has been reported to improve heightened mental clarity and focus potentially due to the body's use of ketones as an energy source.
- **Increased resilience:** Fasting may help the body adapt to stress and improve resilience.

- **Better sleep:** Some studies suggest that fasting can improve sleep quality and duration.

In conclusion, fasting is a dynamic process that orchestrates a symphony of physiological and psychological changes within the body. From hormonal regulation to cellular repair, the benefits extend far beyond simple caloric restriction. Understanding these intricacies empowers individuals to harness the potential of fasting for improved metabolic health, longevity, and cognitive function.

Different Methods of Intermittent Fasting

Embarking on the journey of intermittent fasting is a profound exploration of the body's natural rhythm and its response to periods of nourishment and abstention. Let's delve into the different methods of intermittent fasting and unravel the science that underpins its transformative effects.

16/8 Method:

The 16/8 method, also known as the Leangains protocol or time-restricted eating, involves fasting for 16 hours and eating within an 8-hour window. This method is popular because it aligns seamlessly with the natural circadian rhythm, optimizing metabolic processes; is easy to follow and can be incorporated into most lifestyles. During the fasting period, you can drink water, coffee, or other non-caloric beverages.

5:2 Method:

In the 5:2 method, individuals consume a regular diet for five days a week and limit caloric intake to around 500-600 calories on the remaining two non-consecutive days. This approach provides a balance between intermittent fasting and a more traditional eating pattern. This method is flexible and can be adjusted to fit individual needs.

Alternate-Day Fasting:

As the name suggests, alternate-day fasting involves alternating between days of regular eating and days of significant caloric restriction or fasting. This method offers flexibility, allowing individuals to choose fasting days that align with their schedule and lifestyle. This method can be challenging for some individuals, but it has been shown to be effective for weight loss and improving metabolic health.

Warrior Diet:

Inspired by ancient warrior cultures, this method involves consuming small amounts of raw fruits and vegetables during the day and indulging in a large, satisfying meal at night. The Warrior Diet emphasizes undereating during the day and feasting during a specific eating window. This method is based on the idea that humans evolved to eat one large meal at the end of the day, and it can be effective for weight loss and improving metabolic health.

Eat-Stop-Eat

This entails fasting for a full 24 hours once or twice a week. It's crucial to choose days that align with your schedule and preferences.

The Science Behind Intermittent Fasting

Intermittent fasting has been shown to have various metabolic, hormonal, and cellular effects on the body.

1. Metabolic Changes: Intermittent fasting leads to increased fat oxidation, ketosis, and autophagy, which can promote weight loss and overall health. It can also improve insulin sensitivity, which can be beneficial for individuals with diabetes or prediabetes.

These metabolic adaptations extend beyond simple calorie restriction. As the body transitions from the fed to the fasting state, insulin levels drop, prompting the utilization of stored glycogen and, subsequently, fat for energy. This metabolic flexibility contributes to weight management and overall metabolic health.

2. Hormonal Impact:

Hormones play a pivotal role in orchestrating the effects of intermittent fasting. Insulin sensitivity improves, aiding in blood sugar regulation and reducing the risk of type 2 diabetes. Growth hormone levels rise, facilitating fat burning and muscle preservation. Additionally, intermittent fasting has been linked to increased norepinephrine and brain-derived neurotrophic factor (BDNF), influencing mood and cognitive function.

Intermittent fasting can affect several hormones in the body, including insulin, growth hormone, and cortisol. These hormonal changes can promote fat loss, muscle gain, and overall health.

3. Cellular Repair and Longevity:

Intermittent fasting triggers a cellular repair process known as autophagy, wherein cells remove damaged components, promoting renewal and longevity. This cleansing process contributes to the prevention of various age-related diseases and supports overall cellular health.

In essence, intermittent fasting is not just a dietary approach; it's a lifestyle that taps into the body's innate ability to adapt and thrive. By understanding the different methods and the science behind intermittent fasting, individuals can tailor their approach to align with personal preferences and health goals.

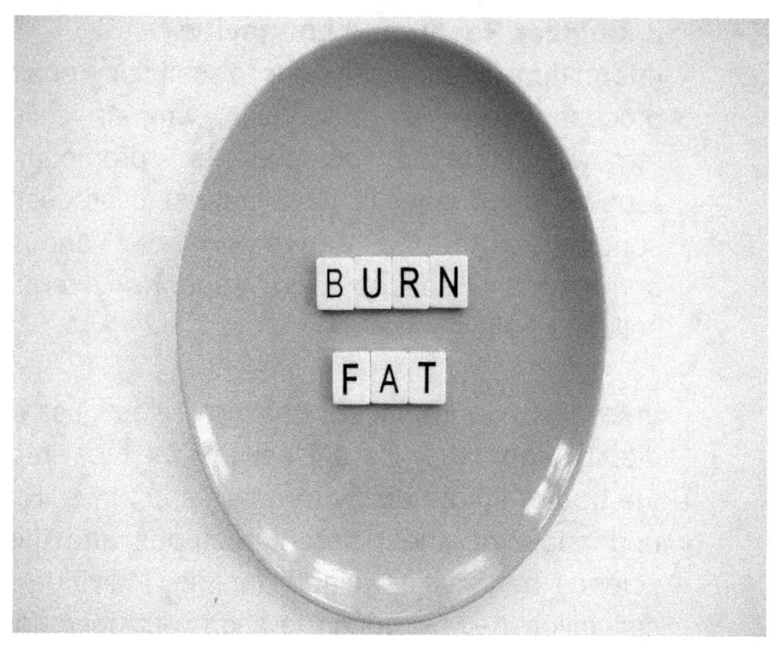

BURN
FAT

CHAPTER ONE

CUSTOMISING INTERMITTENT FASTING FOR WOMEN OVER 50

Hormonal Changes and Menopause

Hormonal changes and menopause can significantly impact women over 50. During menopause, the body undergoes major hormonal shifts, with a decrease in estrogen and progesterone levels. These changes can lead to symptoms such as hot flashes, night sweats, and mood swing. Additionally, the decline in testosterone, which begins years before menopause, may affect libido and sexual health. The menopausal transition is characterized by a significant decline in reproductive hormones, particularly estrogen, which can cause various symptoms and health effects.

It's important to address these hormonal changes. Understanding the impact of these changes on metabolism and overall health is crucial for developing and adopting a well tailored intermittent fasting plan to support the well-being of women in this age group.

Impact on Metabolism

Hormonal changes and menopause can have a significant impact on metabolism in women over 50. During menopause, there is a decrease in estrogen and progesterone levels, which can lead to dysregulated lipid metabolism, visceral fat accumulation, and altered fatty acid metabolism. Menopausal transition is also associated with significant weight gain, an increase in abdominal adiposity, and a decrease in energy expenditure. These changes can contribute to metabolic disorders such as dyslipidemia, impaired glucose tolerance, insulin resistance, hyperinsulinemia, and type 2 diabete.

The decline in estrogen levels during menopause can also lead to unfavorable changes in blood glucose levels, as estrogen is known to enhance insulin sensitivity and glucose disposal in women. Additionally, menopausal women are more likely to experience metabolic syndrome and cardiovascular risk factors.

Addressing hormonal imbalances

Menopause often comes with its own set of challenges, including hormonal imbalances that may affect mood, energy levels, and overall well-being. Addressing these hormonal imbalances in women over 50 is crucial for their overall health and well-being. Since hormonal imbalances can lead to discomfort and health issues, there are manageable elements that can influence hormone levels. Some strategies to address hormonal imbalances include:

Diet: A balanced and healthy diet can play a significant role in addressing hormonal imbalances. Certain foods, such as dairy products, may impact hormone levels, so being wary of their consumption can be beneficial. Within these pages, the cookbook transforms into a supportive guide, offering recipes curated to nourish and support hormonal balance. From ingredients known to alleviate symptoms to thoughtful considerations within the fasting routine, it becomes a trusted resource for addressing both the physical and emotional dimensions of hormonal changes.

Stress Management: Chronic/severe stress can contribute to hormonal imbalances. Implementing stress-reducing techniques such as mindfulness, meditation, or yoga can help manage stress levels and support hormone balance

Sleep: Prioritizing quality sleep is essential for hormonal balance. Getting a full, undisturbed night's rest can help the body regulate hormone levels

Exercise: Regular physical activity is important for overall health and can also contribute to hormone balance. Incorporating exercise into the daily routine can help manage hormone

Essential nutrients for women over 50.

As a woman over 50, it's essential to pay attention to your nutritional needs to support your health and well-being. This cookbook is a culinary compass, guiding women towards recipes rich in calcium for bone health, heart-friendly ingredients, and a spectrum of vitamins and minerals essential for overall vitality. It isn't just about meals; but about crafting a dietary approach that comprehensively nourishes the body during this significant life stage.

Here are some key nutrients that are particularly important for women in this age group:

Calcium for bone health

Calcium is crucial for maintaining bone strength, especially after menopause, when the risk of osteoporosis increases. Good food sources of calcium include dairy products, leafy greens, and fortified foods.

Vitamin D

This vitamin is important for calcium absorption and bone health. It also plays a role in muscle function and immune health. Sunlight, fatty fish, and fortified foods are good sources of vitamin D.

Vitamin B12

This vitamin is also essential for nerve function and the production of red blood cells. As we age, our ability to absorb vitamin B12 may decrease, so it's important to ensure an adequate intake through foods like meat, fish, and fortified cereals.

Protein for muscle preservation

Protein is important for maintaining muscle mass and overall health. Great sources of protein may include lean meats, poultry, fish, eggs, dairy, legumes, and nuts.

Fiber

Fiber is important for digestive health and can help with managing weight and reducing the risk of certain diseases. Fruits, vegetables, whole grains, legumes, and nuts are all good sources of fiber.

Potassium

Potassium is important for heart health and muscle function. Good food sources of potassium include fruits, vegetables, and legumes.

In addition to obtaining these nutrients from a balanced diet, it's also recommended to take a daily multivitamin for your age group and to consider incorporating foods rich in these essential nutrients into your meals. By paying attention to these key nutrients, you can support your overall health and well-being as you navigate this stage of life.

Adequate caloric intake

As women age, their caloric needs change due to factors such as metabolic changes and changes in body composition. For women over 50, moderately active individuals may require approximately 1,800 calories per day to maintain weight, and around 1,300 to 1,700 calories per day to lose weight. It's important to pay special attention to the intake of specific nutrients such as calcium, vitamin D, protein, and B vitamins. The Mediterranean, flexitarian DASH, and MIND diets are recommended for women over 50, but the best diet is the one that can be followed long-term and makes you feel your best. Small, incremental changes to the diet can also provide significant health benefits. Before making any major changes to your diet or adding supplements, it's advisable to consult a healthcare provider to ensure it aligns with your needs. Additionally, it's important to focus on whole, minimally processed foods and to maintain a balanced eating pattern that emphasizes key nutrients.

Micronutrient considerations

Micronutrient Considerations play a pivotal role in promoting optimal health and well-being, especially for women over the age of 50. As our bodies undergo natural physiological changes, addressing specific nutritional needs becomes paramount to support overall vitality.

To embark on this journey, it is crucial to underscore the significance of calcium intake. Postmenopausal women often contend with reduced bone density, making adequate calcium consumption imperative to mitigate the risk of osteoporosis. Incorporating fortified plant-based dairy alternatives, and leafy greens into your diet ensures a robust foundation for bone health.

> Transitioning seamlessly to another key micronutrient, vitamin D deserves special attention. Often dubbed the "sunshine vitamin," vitamin D aids in calcium absorption, further fortifying bone integrity. In the absence of sufficient sunlight exposure, consider incorporating fatty fish, fortified cereals, and vitamin D supplements to maintain optimal levels.

> Iron is another element critical for maintaining energy levels and preventing anemia. Postmenopausal women should strike a balance in iron consumption, as excessive intake may pose health risks. Include lean meats, legumes, and fortified cereals in your diet to meet iron requirements judiciously.

> The journey through menopause may also underscore the significance of maintaining cardiovascular health.

Omega-3 fatty acids, found abundantly in fatty fish like salmon and walnuts, prove instrumental in supporting heart function. Including these sources in your diet contributes to a heart-healthy regimen, crucial for women navigating the nuances of this life stage.

➢ Additionally, the role of antioxidants cannot be overstated. Vitamins C and E, coupled with selenium, act as formidable allies against oxidative stress. Incorporate citrus fruits, nuts, seeds, and whole grains to harness the protective power of antioxidants, safeguarding your cells from the wear and tear of aging.

➢ In the realm of micronutrient considerations, the B-vitamins stand out for their multifaceted contributions. Vitamin B12, in particular, becomes pivotal as absorption diminishes with age. Fortified foods and supplements offer viable solutions to bridge the nutritional gap and sustain cognitive function.

In summary, embracing a well-rounded diet that addresses specific micronutrient needs is integral to supporting the health and vitality of women over 50. Calcium, vitamin D, iron, omega-3 fatty acids, antioxidants, and B-vitamins collectively weave a tapestry of nutritional support, empowering you to navigate this phase of life with resilience and optimal well-being. Remember, these dietary adjustments are not merely a choice but a proactive step toward embracing the best version of yourself.

CHAPTER TWO

GETTING STARTED WITH INTERMITTENT FASTING

Embarking on the journey of intermittent fasting demands a mindful approach, integrating both mental and physical preparations. Below, are the nuanced steps to seamlessly initiate this transformative practice.

A. Preparing Mentally and Physically

Setting Realistic Goals

Before diving into intermittent fasting, establish clear and attainable objectives tailored to your lifestyle. Begin with a realistic timeframe for fasting intervals, considering your daily routine and personal preferences. Setting achievable goals not only fosters a positive mindset but also ensures sustainable adherence to this dietary regimen.

Transitioning into intermittent fasting is a gradual process, and defining milestones provides a structured pathway. Whether aiming for weight management, improved metabolism, or enhanced mental clarity, align your goals with your broader health aspirations.

Consulting with Healthcare Professionals
Seeking guidance from healthcare professionals is a crucial step in ensuring the compatibility of intermittent fasting with your individual health profile. Schedule a consultation with your doctor to discuss any existing medical conditions, medications, or dietary restrictions. This proactive approach ensures that intermittent fasting aligns seamlessly with your overall well-being.

B. Creating a Fasting Schedule

Finding the Fasting Pattern That's Perfect for You

When it comes to finding the right fasting pattern for you, it's essential to assess your individual needs and goals.

Are you aiming for weight management, improved metabolic function, or enhanced mental clarity? Understanding your aspirations provides a compass for selecting a fasting pattern tailored to your objectives.

There are several popular intermittent fasting methods, each with its own pros and cons. One common approach is time-restricted eating, such as the 16/8 method, which involves fasting for 16 hours and eating within an 8-hour window. Another method is the 5:2 diet, which allows for normal eating for 5 days a week and restricts calorie intake on the other 2 days. Eat Stop Eat involves a 24-hour fast once or twice per week, while alternate-day fasting alternates between fasting and non-fasting days.

To choose the right fasting pattern, it's important to consider your comfort level during the fasts. If you experience excessive discomfort, it may be a sign that the fasting protocol needs adjusting. Start with a 12-hour fast and gradually scale up to find a program that works best for your body. It's also crucial to consult a healthcare professional before making any drastic changes to your diet, especially if you have a history of eating disorders.

Ultimately, the key to success with intermittent fasting is to find a pattern that aligns with your lifestyle and is sustainable for you. It's not a one-size-fits-all approach, so it may take some trial and error to determine the best fit for your individual needs and goals. Always prioritize your health and well-being when exploring fasting patterns.

Gradual Transition into Intermittent Fasting

Transitioning into intermittent fasting is most effective when approached gradually. Initiate the process by extending the time between meals, allowing your body to adapt to longer periods without food. Begin with a modest fasting window and gradually increase it as your body adjusts.

This incremental approach minimizes the risk of feeling overwhelmed and enhances the likelihood of sustainable adherence. Acknowledge that intermittent fasting is a personalized journey, and the pace of transition should resonate with your comfort level.

In essence, getting started with intermittent fasting is a holistic endeavor that encompasses mental fortitude, realistic goal-setting, informed consultations, and a tailored fasting schedule. By prioritizing these foundational steps, you pave the way for a seamless and sustainable integration of intermittent fasting into your lifestyle, fostering a journey toward enhanced well-being and vitality.

Frequently Asked Questions

Intermittent fasting (IF) has become popular for weight loss, health improvement, and simplifying lifestyles. Navigating the realm of intermittent fasting often sparks a multitude of questions and concerns. Let's delve into some of the frequently asked questions, then, address some common misconceptions, and provide clear, concise answers to guide you through this transformative journey.

Common Questions and Concerns about Intermittent Fasting

Can I drink liquids during the fast?
Yes, you can drink water, tea, coffee, and other non-caloric beverages during the fast.

Is it unhealthy to skip breakfast?
No, skipping breakfast is not unhealthy. Intermittent fasting has been shown to have many benefits for the body and brain.

Will I Experience Nutrient Deficiencies?
It's understandable to worry about nutrient intake during fasting periods. However, with a well-balanced diet during eating windows, incorporating a variety of nutrient-rich foods, deficiencies are unlikely. Consulting a

healthcare professional can further alleviate concerns.

Can I Exercise During Fasting?

Absolutely. In fact, many individuals find that light to moderate exercise during fasting enhances the benefits. Hydration is key, and scheduling workouts during eating windows can optimize performance.

Is Intermittent Fasting Suitable for Everyone?

While generally safe, it's crucial to consult with a healthcare professional before starting intermittent fasting, especially for individuals with underlying health conditions, pregnant or breastfeeding women, and those on certain medications.

Is there a 'right way' to fast?

Intermittent fasting is less about what you eat and more about when you eat. There are different methods, such as the 16:8 method, the 5:2 diet etc.

Will Fasting Slow Down My Metabolism?

Contrary to a common misconception, intermittent fasting may actually support metabolic health. Studies suggest that it can enhance metabolic flexibility, encouraging the body to efficiently switch between burning glucose and fat for energy.

How Soon Will I See Results?
 - Results vary from person to person. But many individuals notice changes within a few weeks. Factors like consistency, diet quality, and individual metabolism play a role. Patience and consistency are key.

What Can I Eat During Eating Windows?
- Emphasize nutrient-dense foods: lean proteins, fruits, vegetables, whole grains, and healthy fats. Prioritize a well-balanced diet to maximize the benefits of intermittent fasting.

Addressing Misconceptions

Myth: Fasting slows down your metabolism. -There is currently no evidence to suggest that fasting causes a significant slowdown in metabolism.
Myth: Fasting causes nutrient deficiencies.
- Fasting may positively impact nutrient absorption and improve how the body uses nutrients.
Myth: IF is unhealthy and leads to starvation mode.

-When followed correctly with healthy eating options, intermittent fasting can be beneficial for weight loss.

Myth: Fasting Leads to Muscle Loss
- Intermittent fasting, when coupled with adequate protein intake, is not associated with significant muscle loss. In fact, it may contribute to muscle preservation by promoting growth hormone release.

Myth: You Must Follow a Strict Eating Window
- Flexibility is a key principle of intermittent fasting. While structured eating windows provide guidance, it's essential to find a rhythm that suits your lifestyle. Adaptability promotes long-term adherence.

In conclusion, addressing frequently asked questions about intermittent fasting involves dispelling common concerns, clarifying misconceptions, and providing practical guidance. By understanding the nuances of this transformative approach, you can embark on your intermittent fasting journey with confidence, armed with knowledge to optimize your well-being.

CHAPTER THREE

NUTRIENT-DENSE FOODS FOR WOMEN OVER 50

As women navigate the unique nutritional needs that accompany the age of 50 and beyond, prioritizing nutrient-dense foods becomes paramount. Incorporating these foods into daily meals contributes to overall health and supports specific concerns related to aging.

Key Nutrient-Dense and Fast Friendly Foods/drinks:

Navigating intermittent fasting successfully involves choosing foods that complement fasting periods. Fast-friendly options help sustain energy levels and provide essential nutrients, ensuring a balanced approach to this dietary regimen.

Calcium-Rich Sources:
Counteract bone density loss with dairy, fortified plant-based alternatives, and leafy greens.

Fiber-Packed Foods:
Enhance digestive health and manage weight with whole grains, legumes, and a variety of fruits and vegetables.

Lean Proteins:
Support muscle health and metabolism with lean meats, poultry, fish, eggs, and plant-based protein sources.

Omega-3 Fatty Acids:
Promote heart health and cognitive function through fatty fish, flaxseeds, chia seeds, and walnuts.

Antioxidant-Rich Options:
Combat oxidative stress with colorful fruits, vegetables, nuts, and seeds, aiding in cell protection.

Low-Glycemic Fruits:
Include berries, apples, or pears for a natural energy boost without causing rapid blood sugar spikes.

Vegetables:
- Incorporate non-starchy vegetables like leafy greens, broccoli, and bell peppers to maintain fiber intake.

Nuts and Seeds:
Provide healthy fats and a satisfying crunch, contributing to satiety during fasting windows.

Hydrating Beverages:
Prioritize water, herbal teas, and black coffee to stay hydrated and support appetite control.

Meal Planning Tips

Below, are the tips to consider when planning your meals on intermittent fasting.

Creating a Meal Plan

Crafting a thoughtful meal plan ensures that nutrient needs are met while aligning with intermittent fasting goals. Consider these steps to tailor a meal plan to your lifestyle:

Establish Fasting Windows

Define your fasting and eating windows to structure your daily meals effectively.

Balance Macronutrients

Include a mix of proteins, carbohydrates, and healthy fats to promote overall nutritional balance.

Incorporate Variety

Ensure a diverse range of foods to obtain a spectrum of vitamins and minerals essential for well-being.

Tips for a Successful Intermittent Fasting

Stay Hydrated:

Prioritize water intake to support overall health and help manage hunger during fasting periods.

Gradual Transition:

Ease into intermittent fasting, gradually extending fasting windows to allow the body to adapt.

Listen to Your Body:

- Pay attention to hunger cues and adjust your eating windows or food choices accordingly.

CHAPTER FOUR

NUTRIENT-DENSE BREAKFAST OPTIONS

Protein-Packed Quinoa Breakfast Bowl

- **Preparation Time**: 25 minutes
- **Yield**: 2 servings
- **Caloric Count**: Approximately 350 calories per serving
- **Nutritional Information per Serving**:
 - Protein: 20g
 - Fiber: 8g
 - Calcium: 15% of DV
 - Iron: 20% of DV

- **Ingredients**:
 - 1/2 cup quinoa
 - 1 cup almond milk
 - 1/4 tsp cinnamon
 - 1/2 cup mixed berries
 - 2 tbsp chopped nuts
 - 1 tbsp maple syrup or honey

- **Method of Preparation:**
 1. Rinse quinoa and cook with almond milk and cinnamon until fluffy.
 2. Divide the cooked quinoa into bowls and top with mixed berries, nuts, and a drizzle of honey or maple syrup.

- **Substitutes**:
 - Quinoa: Buckwheat or amaranth
 - Almond milk: Oat milk or soy milk
 - Mixed berries: Sliced banana or diced apple
- Health Benefits: Quinoa is rich in protein and fiber, which can help manage weight and support bone health.

Chia Seed Pudding

- **Preparation Time:** 10 minutes (+overnight chilling)
- **Yield**: 2 servings
- **Caloric Count:** Approximately 280 calories per serving
- **Nutritional Information per Serving**:
 - Omega-3: 5g
 - Calcium: 20% of DV
 - Magnesium: 15% of DV
 - Iron: 10% of DV

- **Ingredients**:
 - 1/4 cup chia seeds

- 1 cup coconut milk
- 1/2 tsp vanilla extract
- 1 tbsp agave nectar or honey
- Sliced fruits for topping

- **Method of Preparation:**
1. In a bowl, mix chia seeds, coconut milk, vanilla extract, and sweetener. Leave it for over 5 minutes, then stir again.
2. Cover and refrigerate overnight.
3. In the morning, divide the pudding into serving glasses and top with sliced fruits.
- Substitutes:
 - Coconut milk: Almond milk or cashew milk
 - Honey: Maple syrup or stevia

- **Health Benefits**: Chia seeds are a great source of omega-3 fatty acids, which can help support heart health and reduce inflammation.

Green Smoothie

- **Preparation Time**: 10 minutes
- **Yield**: 2 servings
- **Caloric Count:** Approximately 200 calories per serving
- **Nutritional Information per Serving**:
 - Vitamin C: 90% of DV
 - Vitamin K: 80% of DV
 - Folate: 30% of DV

- Fiber: 6g

- **Ingredients**:
 - 2 cups spinach
 - 1 cup kale
 - 1 green apple, cored
 - 1/2 cucumber
 - 1/2 lemon, juiced
 - 1 cup coconut water

- **Method of Preparation:**
 1. Blend all the ingredients until smooth.
 2. Add more coconut water if needed for desired consistency.
- Substitutes:
 - Spinach: Swiss chard or arugula
 - Kale: Romaine lettuce or parsley
 - Green apple: Pear or kiwi

- **Health Benefits:** Green leafy vegetables are rich in vitamin K, which is important for bone health and may help reduce the risk of fractures in postmenopausal women.

Flaxseed and Berry Breakfast Parfait

- **Preparation Time**: 15 minutes
- **Yield**: 2 servings
- **Caloric Count**: Approximately 320 calories per serving

- **Nutritional Information per Serving:**
 - Omega-3: 3g
 - Protein: 15g
 - Fiber: 10g
 - Calcium: 20% of DV

- **Ingredients**:
 - 1 cup Greek yogurt
 - 2 tbsp ground flaxseeds
 - 1 cup mixed berries
 - 1/4 cup granola

- **Method of Preparation:**
 1. In serving glasses, layer Greek yogurt, ground flaxseeds, mixed berries, and granola.
 2. Repeat the layers.

- **Substitutes**:
 - Greek yogurt: Dairy-free yogurt or cottage cheese
 - Ground flaxseeds: Chia seeds or hemp hearts

- **Health Benefits:** Flaxseeds are rich in lignans, which have been shown to have potential benefits for menopausal women, including reducing the frequency and severity of hot flashes.

Cinnamon-Spiced Baked Apple Oatmeal

- **Preparation Time**: 30 minutes
- **Yield**: 4 servings
- **Caloric Count**: Approximately 280 calories per serving
- **Nutritional Information per Serving**:
 - Fiber: 7g
 - Vitamin C: 10% of DV
 - Iron: 15% of DV
 - Calcium: 10% of DV

- **Ingredients**:
 - 2 cups rolled oats
 - 2 1/2 cups almond milk
 - 2 apples, diced
 - 2 tbsp maple syrup
 - 1 tsp cinnamon

- **Method of Preparation:**
 1. Set the oven temperature to 375°F (190°C).
 2. In a baking dish, combine rolled oats, almond milk, diced apples, maple syrup, and cinnamon.
 3. Bake for 25-30 minutes until the oats are tender and the top is golden.

- **Substitutes**:
 - Almond milk: Oat milk or soy milk

- Maple syrup: Honey or agave nectar

- **Health Benefits:** Apples are a good source of soluble fiber, which can help support healthy cholesterol levels and aid in digestion.

Tips:
- To save time, prepare the ingredients the night before and assemble the recipes in the morning.
- Experiment with different fruits, nuts, and seeds to keep the recipes exciting and varied.
- Incorporate a variety of colorful ingredients to ensure a wide range of nutrients and health benefits.

Quinoa Power Bowl

Preparation Time: 30 minutes
Yield: 4 servings
Caloric Count: Approximately 350 calories per serving

Ingredients:
- 1 cup quinoa, cooked
- 1 cup kale, chopped
- 1/2 cup sweet potatoes, cubed
- 1/4 cup feta cheese, crumbled
- 2 tablespoons olive oil
- Salt and pepper to taste

Method of Preparation:
1. Roast sweet potatoes in olive oil until golden.
2. Mix quinoa, kale, and roasted sweet potatoes.
3. Top with crumbled feta and season with salt and pepper.

Health Benefits:
- Quinoa contains phytoestrogens, aiding hormonal balance.
- Kale offers calcium for bone health during menopause.

Substitutes:
- Swap sweet potatoes with butternut squash.

Tips:
- Add a squeeze of lemon for extra flavor.

Salmon Avocado Toast

Preparation Time: 20 minutes
Yield: 2 servings
Caloric Count: Approximately 400 calories per serving

Ingredients:
- 2 slices whole-grain bread

- 1 avocado, mashed
- 150g smoked salmon
- 1 tablespoon lemon juice
- Dill for garnish

Method of Preparation:
1. Toast the bread slices to your preference.
2. Spread mashed avocado on each slice.
3. Top with smoked salmon, drizzle with lemon juice, and garnish with dill.

Health Benefits:
- Salmon provides omega-3 fatty acids, essential for hormonal health.
- Avocado offers monounsaturated fats, promoting heart health.

Substitutes:
- Use gluten-free bread if needed.

Tips:
- Opt for wild-caught salmon for optimal omega-3 content.

Turmeric Golden Oatmeal

Preparation Time: 25 minutes
Yield: 3 servings
Caloric Count: Approximately 320 calories per serving

Ingredients:
- 1 cup rolled oats
- 2 cups almond milk
- 1 teaspoon turmeric
- 1/2 teaspoon cinnamon
- 1 tablespoon maple syrup
- 1/4 cup chopped walnuts

Method of Preparation:
1. Cook oats in almond milk with turmeric and cinnamon.
2. Sweeten with maple syrup and top with chopped walnuts.

Health Benefits:
- Turmeric has anti-inflammatory properties, easing menopausal symptoms.
- Almond milk is a calcium-rich dairy alternative.

Substitutes:
- Use any nut butter instead of walnuts.

Tips:
- Sprinkle flaxseeds for an extra boost of omega-3.

Sweet Potato and Spinach Frittata

Preparation Time: 45 minutes
Yield: 4 servings
Caloric Count: Approximately 250 calories per serving

Ingredients:
1 large sweet potato, peeled and grated
2 cups fresh spinach, chopped
1 onion, diced
6 eggs
1/4 cup feta cheese, crumbled
2 tablespoons olive oil
Salt and pepper to taste

Method of Preparation:
Preheat oven to 375°F (190°C).
In a skillet, sauté grated sweet potato, spinach, and diced onion in olive oil until softened.
Then in a bowl, beat the eggs and season with salt and pepper.
Pour eggs over the sweet potato mixture, sprinkle with feta cheese, and bake for 25-30 minutes.

Health Benefits:
Sweet potatoes offer beta-carotene, beneficial for skin health.

Spinach is rich in iron, addressing potential menopausal fatigue.
Substitutes:
Use goat cheese instead of feta.
Tips:
Add a pinch of turmeric for anti-inflammatory properties.

Salmon and Avocado Breakfast Wrap

Preparation Time: 20 minutes
Yield: 2 servings
Caloric Count: Approximately 350 calories per serving

Ingredients:
2 whole-grain wraps
1/2 lb smoked salmon
1 avocado, sliced
4 eggs, scrambled
1 tablespoon cream cheese
Fresh dill for garnish
Salt and pepper to taste

Method of Preparation:
Spread cream cheese on each wrap.
Layer with smoked salmon, sliced avocado, and scrambled eggs.
Season with salt, pepper, and garnish with fresh dill before rolling.

Health Benefits:
Salmon provides omega-3 fatty acids, supporting heart and brain health.
Avocado offers healthy monounsaturated fats.

Substitutes:
Use whole-grain toast instead of wraps.

Tips:
You can sprinkle with chia seeds for an extra nutrient boost.

Greek Yogurt Parfait with Granola and Berries

Preparation Time: 15 minutes
Yield: 2 servings
Caloric Count: Approximately 200 calories per serving

Ingredients:
1 cup Greek yogurt
1/2 cup granola (preferably low-sugar)
1/2 cup mixed berries (strawberries, blueberries)
1 tablespoon honey

Method of Preparation:
In a glass, layer Greek yogurt, and then granola, with mixed berries.
Repeat the layers.
Drizzle with honey before serving.

Health Benefits:
Greek yogurt provides probiotics for gut health. Berries offer antioxidants that support overall well-being.

Substitutes:
Use maple syrup instead of honey.

Tips:
For added fiber, add a sprinkle of chia seeds.

Almond Butter and Banana Overnight Oats

Preparation Time: 10 minutes (plus overnight soaking)
Yield: 2 servings
Caloric Count: Approximately 280 calories per serving

Ingredients:
1 cup rolled oats
1 cup almond milk
2 tablespoons almond butter

1 banana, sliced
1 tablespoon chia seeds
1 tablespoon honey

Method of Preparation:
In a jar, combine rolled oats, almond milk, almond butter, banana slices, and chia seeds.
Stir well, cover, and refrigerate overnight.
Drizzle with honey before serving.

Health Benefits:
Oats provide complex carbohydrates for sustained energy.
Almond butter offers healthy fats and protein.

Substitutes:
Use peanut butter instead of almond butter.

Tips:
Top with sliced almonds for added crunch.

Turmeric and Ginger Smoothie

Preparation Time: 10 minutes
Yield: 2 servings
Caloric Count: Approximately 180 calories per serving

Ingredients:
1 cup coconut milk

1 banana, frozen
1/2 teaspoon turmeric powder
1/2 teaspoon ginger, grated
1 tablespoon chia seeds
Ice cubes

Method of Preparation:
Blend coconut milk, frozen banana, turmeric powder, grated ginger, and chia seeds until smooth.
Add ice cubes and blend again for a refreshing texture.

Health Benefits:
Turmeric has anti-inflammatory properties that may help with menopausal symptoms.
Ginger may alleviate nausea and aid digestion.

Substitutes:
Use almond milk instead of coconut milk.

Tips:
Add a squeeze of lemon for a zesty twist.

Egg and Veggie Breakfast Skillet

Preparation Time: 25 minutes
Yield: 2 servings
Caloric Count: Approximately 280 calories per serving

Ingredients:
4 eggs
1 cup cherry tomatoes, halved
1/2 cup bell peppers, diced
1/2 cup spinach, chopped
1 tablespoon olive oil
Salt and pepper to taste
Fresh herbs for garnish

Method of Preparation:
In a skillet, heat olive oil and sauté cherry tomatoes, bell peppers, and spinach until wilted.
Crack eggs into the skillet, season with salt and pepper, and cook until the whites are set.
Garnish with fresh herbs before serving.

Health Benefits:
Eggs include high-quality protein, which is essential for muscle health.
Spinach is rich in iron and other nutrients.

Substitutes:
Use kale instead of spinach.

Tips:
Top with a sprinkle of nutritional yeast for a cheesy flavor.

Cauliflower and Kale Breakfast Hash

Preparation Time: 30 minutes
Yield: 4 servings
Caloric Count: Approximately 220 calories per serving

Ingredients:
2 cups cauliflower rice
2 cups kale, chopped
1 onion, diced
2 cloves garlic, minced
2 tablespoons olive oil
4 eggs
Salt and pepper to taste

Method of Preparation:
Heat the olive oil in a skillet and sauté the onion and garlic until tender.
Cook until the cauliflower rice and kale are soft.
Make wells in the mixture and crack the eggs into each one.
Cook, covered, until the eggs are done to your taste.

Health Benefits:
Cauliflower provides a low-carb alternative to traditional hash.
Kale is rich in vitamins A, C, and K.
Substitutes:

Use broccoli instead of cauliflower.

Tips:
Sprinkle with flaxseeds for added fiber.

Mango and Coconut Chia Pudding

Preparation Time: 15 minutes (plus chilling time)
Yield: 2 servings
Caloric Count: Approximately 220 calories per serving

Ingredients:
1/4 cup chia seeds
1 cup coconut milk
1 tablespoon honey
1 mango, diced
Shredded coconut for garnish

Method of Preparation:
Combine the chia seeds, coconut milk, and honey in a mixing dish.
Refrigerate for at least four hours, and preferably overnight.
Layer with diced mango and garnish with shredded coconut before serving.

Health Benefits:

Chia seeds are highly abundant in omega-3 fatty acids and fiber.
Mango provides vitamins A and C for immune support.

Substitutes:
Use almond milk instead of coconut milk.

Tips:
Top with a dollop of Greek yogurt for creaminess.

Blueberry and Almond Smoothie Bowl

Preparation Time: 15 minutes
Yield: 2 servings
Caloric Count: Approximately 250 calories per serving

Ingredients:
1 cup frozen blueberries
1 banana, frozen
1/2 cup almond milk
1/4 cup almonds, chopped
2 tablespoons Greek yogurt
Granola for topping

Method of Preparation:
Blend frozen blueberries, frozen banana, and almond milk until smooth.
Pour into bowls and top with chopped almonds, Greek yogurt, and granola.

Health Benefits:
Blueberries offer antioxidants that support cognitive function.
Almonds provide healthy fats and vitamin E.

Substitutes:
Use cashew milk instead of almond milk.

Tips:
Drizzle with almond butter for extra richness.

Coconut Flour Pancakes with Mixed Berries

Preparation Time: 20 minutes
Yield: 2 servings
Caloric Count: Approximately 280 calories per serving

Ingredients:
1/2 cup coconut flour
1 teaspoon baking powder
2 eggs
1/2 cup coconut milk

1 tablespoon honey
Mixed berries for topping

Method of Preparation:
In a mixing dish or bowl, whisk together the eggs and season with salt and pepper.
Heat a skillet and spoon batter to make small pancakes.
Cook until bubbles form, flip, and cook the other side.
Top with mixed berries before serving.

Health Benefits:
Coconut flour is a gluten-free alternative rich in fiber.
Berries offer antioxidants that support overall well-being.

Substitutes:
Use almond flour instead of coconut flour.

Tips:
Serve with a dollop of coconut cream.

Spinach and Feta Omelette

Preparation Time: 15 minutes
Yield: 2 servings
Caloric Count: Approximately 230 calories per serving

Ingredients:
4 eggs
1 cup fresh spinach, chopped
1/4 cup feta cheese, crumbled
1/2 onion, diced
1 tablespoon olive oil
Salt and pepper to taste

Method of Preparation:
In a bowl or mixing dish, whisk together the eggs and season with salt and pepper.
In a skillet, sauté onion and spinach in olive oil until wilted.
Pour eggs over the spinach mixture, sprinkle with feta, and cook until set.

Health Benefits:
Spinach provides iron and other essential nutrients.
Eggs offer high-quality protein for muscle health.

Substitutes:
Use goat cheese instead of feta.

Tips:
Add cherry tomatoes for a burst of flavor.

Cauliflower and Spinach Breakfast Burrito

Preparation Time: 30 minutes
Yield: 2 servings
Caloric Count: Approximately 320 calories per serving

Ingredients:
2 whole-grain tortillas
1 cup cauliflower rice
1/2 cup black beans, drained and rinsed
2 eggs, scrambled
1/4 cup salsa
Fresh cilantro for garnish

Method of Preparation:
In a pan, sauté cauliflower rice until tender.
Warm tortillas and layer with cauliflower rice, black beans, scrambled eggs, and salsa.
Garnish with fresh cilantro before rolling.

Health Benefits:
Cauliflower is low in calories and high in fiber, supporting weight management.
Black beans provide plant-based protein.

Substitutes:
Use brown rice tortillas for a gluten-free option.

Tips:
Add a slice of avocado for creaminess.

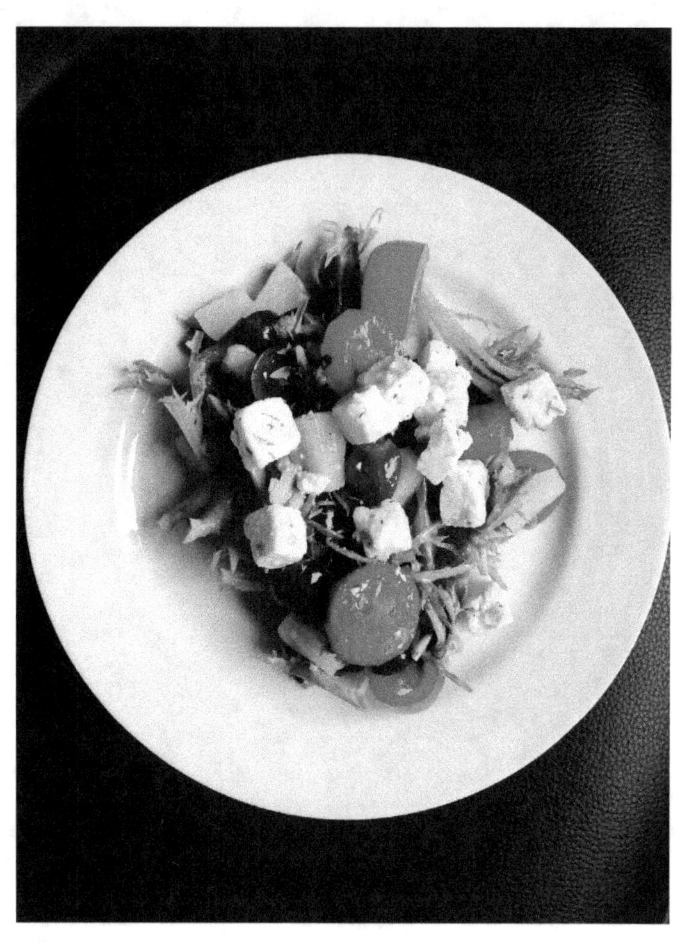

CHAPTER SIX

SALAD RECIPES

Superfood Kale and Quinoa Salad

- **Preparation Time**: 25 minutes
- **Yield**: 4 servings
- **Caloric Count**: Approximately 480 calories per serving
- **Nutritional Information per Serving**:
- Calories: 480
- Total Fat: 24g
- Saturated Fat: (not specified)

- **Ingredients**:
- 1/2 cup dry quinoa, cooked
- 1/2 cup frozen edamame, cooked
- 1/2 bunch curly kale, chopped
- 1/2 cup fresh blueberries
- Other ingredients as desired

- **Method of Preparation**:
1. Cook quinoa and edamame as per package directions.
2. Massage kale with a small amount of olive oil.
3. Combine all ingredients in a large bowl.

4. Add desired dressing, toss well, and serve immediately.

Health Benefits: Kale, quinoa, and edamame are rich in phytonutrients, antioxidants, and essential nutrients, which can help with menopausal issues and hormonal imbalances.

Substitutes:
- Quinoa: Brown rice, couscous, barley
- Edamame: Chickpeas, green peas
- Kale: Spinach, Swiss chard

Tips:
- To minimize bitterness, massage kale with olive oil.
- Prepare the dressing in advance for quicker assembly.

Nutty Spinach and Berry Salad

- **Preparation Time**: 20 minutes
- **Yield**: 4 servings
- **Caloric Count**: Approximately 350 calories per serving
- **Nutritional Information per Serving**:
- Calories: 350
- Total Fat: 18g
- Saturated Fat: (not specified)

- **Ingredients**:
- 6 cups baby spinach
- 1 cup mixed berries
- 1/2 cup mixed nuts (walnuts, almonds)
- Other ingredients as desired

- **Method of Preparation**:
1. Toss baby spinach, mixed berries, and nuts in a large bowl.
2. Drizzle with a light vinaigrette and toss to coat.

Health Benefits: Spinach and berries are rich in vitamins, minerals, and antioxidants, which can support menopausal and hormonal health.

Substitutes:
- Baby spinach: Arugula, kale
- Mixed berries: Sliced apples, pears, dried fruits
- Mixed nuts: Sunflower seeds, pumpkin seeds

Tips:
- Use a light vinaigrette to enhance the flavors without overpowering the salad.
- Toast the mixed nuts for extra crunch and flavor.

Cabbage and Edamame Slaw

- **Preparation Time**: 15 minutes
- **Yield**: 6 servings
- **Caloric Count**: Approximately 250 calories per serving
- **Nutritional Information per Serving:**
- Calories: 250
- Total Fat: 12g
- Saturated Fat: (not specified)

- **Ingredients**:
- 4 cups shredded cabbage
- 1 cup shelled edamame
- 1/2 cup shredded carrots
- Other ingredients as desired

- **Method of Preparation:**
1. In a large bowl, combine shredded cabbage, edamame, and carrots.
2. Toss with a light, tangy dressing.

Health Benefits: Cabbage and edamame are rich in phytonutrients and fiber, which can aid in hormone balance and menopausal symptoms.

Substitutes:
- Shredded cabbage: Shredded Brussels sprouts, kale

- Edamame: Chickpeas, green peas
- Shredded carrots: Sliced radishes, bell peppers

Tips:
- Add a splash of apple cider vinegar to the dressing for a tangy flavor.
- Allow the slaw to marinate for a few hours for enhanced taste.

Mediterranean Chickpea Salad

- **Preparation Time**: 30 minutes
- **Yield**: 4 servings
- **Caloric Count**: Approximately 320 calories per serving
- **Nutritional Information per Serving:**
  - Calories: 320
  - Total Fat: 15g
  - Saturated Fat: (not specified)

- **Ingredients**:
  - 2 cans chickpeas, drained and rinsed
  - 1 cup diced cucumbers
  - 1/2 cup cherry tomatoes, halved
  - Other ingredients as desired

- **Method of Preparation:**
    1. In a large bowl, combine chickpeas, cucumbers, and tomatoes.

2. Toss with a zesty lemon-herb dressing.

Health Benefits: Chickpeas, cucumbers, and tomatoes are rich in plant-based proteins, vitamins, and minerals, which can support menopausal health and hormonal balance.

Substitutes:
- Chickpeas: White beans, black beans
- Diced cucumbers: Diced bell peppers, zucchini
- Cherry tomatoes: Diced Roma tomatoes, sun-dried tomatoes

Tips:
- Prepare the salad in advance to allow the flavors to meld.
- Serve the salad over a bed of leafy greens for added nutrition.

Quinoa and Black Bean Fiesta Salad

- **Preparation Time:** 25 minutes
- **Yield**: 4 servings
- **Caloric Count:** Approximately 380 calories per serving
- **Nutritional Information per Serving:**
  - Calories: 380
  - Total Fat: 20g
  - Saturated Fat: (not specified)

- **Ingredients**:
  - 1 cup cooked quinoa
  - 1 can black beans, drained and rinsed
  - 1/2 cup diced bell peppers
  - Other ingredients as desired

- **Method of Preparation:**
  1. In a large bowl, combine cooked quinoa, black beans, and bell peppers.
  2. Toss with a zesty lime-cilantro dressing.

Health Benefits: Quinoa, black beans, and bell peppers are rich in fiber, vitamins, and minerals, which can aid in hormone regulation and menopausal symptom management.

Substitutes:
- Cooked quinoa: Cooked brown rice, bulgur
- Black beans: Pinto beans, kidney beans
- Diced bell peppers: Diced tomatoes, corn kernels

Tips:
- Add a touch of cumin and chili powder to the dressing for a fiesta-inspired flavor.
- Garnish the salad with fresh cilantro and a squeeze of lime before serving.

Vibrant Veggie Delight Salad

Preparation Time: 20 minutes
Yield: 4 servings
Caloric Count: Approximately 180 calories per serving

Ingredients:
- 2 cups mixed greens (arugula, kale, spinach)
- 1 cup cherry tomatoes, halved
- 1 cucumber, sliced
- 1/2 cup bell peppers, diced
- 1/4 cup pumpkin seeds
- 2 tablespoons balsamic vinaigrette

Method of Preparation:
1. Toss mixed greens, cherry tomatoes, cucumber, and bell peppers in a bowl.
2. Drizzle with balsamic vinaigrette and sprinkle pumpkin seeds.

Health Benefits:
- Leafy greens provide fiber, aiding in digestion during menopause.
- Pumpkin seeds contain zinc, crucial for hormonal balance.

Substitutes:
- Swap balsamic vinaigrette with olive oil and lemon dressing.

Tips:
- For an added protein boost, add grilled chicken.

Quinoa & Chickpea Power Salad

Preparation Time: 30 minutes
Yield: 3 servings
Caloric Count: Approximately 250 calories per serving

Ingredients:
- 1 cup cooked quinoa
- 1 can chickpeas, rinsed and drained
- 1 cup cherry tomatoes, quartered
- 1/2 cup feta cheese, crumbled
- 2 tablespoons olive oil
- 1 teaspoon lemon zest

Method of Preparation:
1. Combine quinoa, chickpeas, cherry tomatoes, and feta cheese in a large bowl.
2. Drizzle with olive oil and sprinkle lemon zest.

Health Benefits:
- Quinoa offers complete protein, vital for muscle health.
- Chickpeas provide fiber and folate, supporting menopausal health.

Substitutes:
- Use goat cheese instead of feta for a tangy twist.

Tips:
- Roast chickpeas for added crunch.

Citrus Bliss Shrimp Salad

Preparation Time: 25 minutes
Yield: 2 servings
Caloric Count: Approximately 220 calories per serving

Ingredients:
- 200g shrimp, cooked and peeled
- 2 cups mixed greens
- 1 grapefruit, segmented
- 1 avocado, sliced
- 2 tablespoons citrus vinaigrette
- Chopped mint for garnish

Method of Preparation:
1. Arrange mixed greens on a plate, top with shrimp, grapefruit segments, and avocado.
2. Drizzle with citrus vinaigrette and garnish with chopped mint.

Health Benefits:
- Shrimp provides iodine, essential for thyroid function.
- Grapefruit contains naringenin, which may help balance hormones.

Substitutes:
- Replace grapefruit with orange segments.

Tips:
- Grilled shrimp adds a smoky flavor.

Mango Tango Quinoa Salad

Preparation Time: 20 minutes
Yield: 4 servings
Caloric Count: Approximately 230 calories per serving

Ingredients:
- 1 cup cooked quinoa
- 1 mango, diced
- 1 cup cucumber, diced
- 1/4 cup red onion, finely chopped
- 1/4 cup cilantro, chopped
- 2 tablespoons lime juice

Method of Preparation:
1. In a bowl, combine quinoa, mango, cucumber, red onion, and cilantro.

2. Drizzle with lime juice and toss gently.

Health Benefits:
- Mango provides vitamin C, aiding collagen production.
- Quinoa offers magnesium, supporting mood during menopause.

Substitutes:
- Substitute cilantro with parsley.

Tips:
- For a spicy kick, you can add a pinch of chili powder

Broccoli Almond Crunch Salad

Preparation Time: 15 minutes
Yield: 3 servings
Caloric Count: Approximately 190 calories per serving

Ingredients:
- 2 cups broccoli florets, blanched
- 1/3 cup almonds, sliced
- 1/4 cup raisins
- 2 tablespoons Greek yogurt
- 1 tablespoon Dijon mustard
- Lemon zest for flavor

Method of Preparation:
1. Mix blanched broccoli, almonds, and raisins in a bowl.
2. In a separate bowl, whisk Greek yogurt, Dijon mustard, and lemon zest.
3. Toss the dressing with the broccoli mixture.

Health Benefits:
- Broccoli contains sulforaphane, linked to lower estrogen levels.
- Almonds offer vitamin E, supporting skin health during menopause.

Substitutes:
- Use dried cranberries instead of raisins.

Tips:
- Let the salad sit for a while to enhance flavors.

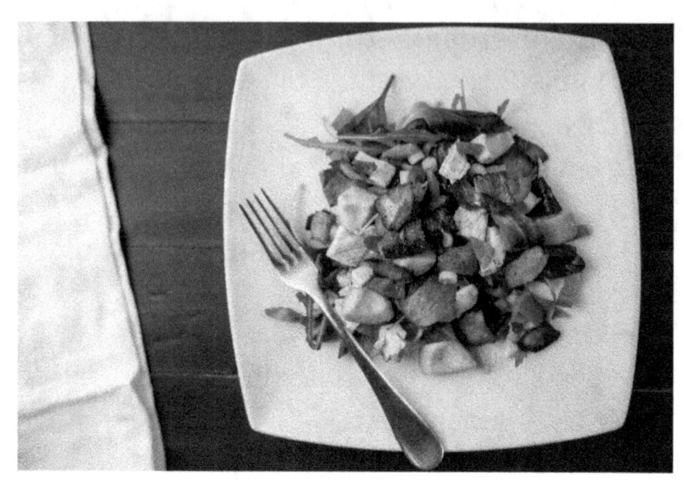

CHAPTER SEVEN

VEGETABLE RECIPES

Broccoli and Cauliflower Salad

- **Preparation Time**: 20 minutes
- **Yield**: 4 servings
- **Caloric count**: 150 calories per serving
- Nutritional information per serving: 6g protein, 10g fat, 10g carbs, 4g fiber

- **Ingredients**:
  - 1 head broccoli, chopped
  - 1 head cauliflower, chopped
  - 1/2 cup chopped red onion
  - 1/2 cup chopped walnuts
  - 1/2 cup dried cranberries
  - 1/4 cup olive oil
  - 2 tbsp apple cider vinegar
  - 1 tbsp honey
  - Salt and pepper to taste

- **Method of Preparation:**
  1. In a large bowl, combine broccoli, cauliflower, red onion, walnuts, and dried cranberries.
  2. In a small bowl, whisk together olive oil, apple cider vinegar, honey, salt, and pepper.

3. Toss the salad along with the dressing to mix.

4. Serve chilled.

Sweet Potato and Black Bean Chili

- **Preparation Time**: 30 minutes
- **Yield**: 6 servings
- **Caloric count**: 250 calories per serving
- Nutritional information per serving: 10g protein, 2g fat, 50g carbs, 15g fiber

- **Ingredients**:
  - 2 sweet potatoes, peeled and diced
  - 1 onion, chopped
  - 2 cloves garlic, minced
  - 1 red bell pepper, chopped
  - 1 can black beans, drained and rinsed
  - 1 can diced tomatoes
  - 2 cups vegetable broth
  - 1 tbsp chili powder
  - 1 tsp cumin
  - Salt and pepper to taste

- **Method of Preparation:**
  1. In a large pot, sauté sweet potatoes, onion, garlic, and red bell pepper until tender.
  2. Add black beans, diced tomatoes, vegetable broth, chili powder, cumin, salt, and pepper.

3. Bring to a boil, then reduce to a low heat and cook for 20 minutes.

4. Serve hot.

Zucchini Noodles with Pesto

- **Preparation Time:** 20 minutes
- **Yield**: 4 servings
- **Caloric Count:** 200 calories per serving
- **Nutritional Information Per Serving:** 5g protein, 15g fat, 10g carbs, 3g fiber

- **Ingredients**:
  - 4 zucchinis, spiralized
  - 1/2 cup pesto
  - 1/4 cup pine nuts
  - Salt and pepper to taste

- **Method Of Preparation:**

1. In a large pan, sauté zucchini noodles until tender.

2. Add pesto and pine nuts, and toss to combine.

3. Season with salt and pepper.

4. Serve hot.

Balsamic Glazed Roasted Brussels Sprouts

- **Preparation Time**: 25 minutes
- **Yield**: 4 servings
- **Caloric Count:** 100 calories per serving
- **Nutritional Information Per Serving:** 4g protein, 5g fat, 15g carbs, 5g fiber

- **Ingredients**:
  - 1 lb of cleaned and cut Brussels sprouts
  - 2 tbsp olive oil
  - Salt and pepper to taste
  - 2 tbsp balsamic vinegar

- **Method Of Preparation:**
  1. Preheat oven to 400°F.
  2. Toss Brussels sprouts with olive oil, salt, and pepper.
  3. Roast for 20 minutes, or until tender and browned.
  4. Drizzle with balsamic vinegar.
  5. Serve hot.

Carrot Ginger Soup

- **Preparation Time:** 30 minutes
- **Yield**: 4 servings
- **Caloric Count:** 150 calories per serving

- **Nutritional Information Per Serving:** 2g protein, 5g fat, 25g carbs, 5g fiber

- **Ingredients**:
  - 1 lb carrots, peeled and chopped
  - 1 onion, chopped
  - 2 cloves garlic, minced
  - 1 tbsp grated ginger
  - 4 cups vegetable broth
  - Salt and pepper to taste

- **Method Of Preparation:**
  1. In a large pot, sauté carrots, onion, garlic, and ginger until tender.
  2. Add vegetable broth, salt, and pepper.
  3. Bring to a boil, then reduce to a low heat and cook for 20 minutes.
  4. Puree the soup until smooth.
  5. Serve hot.

Substitutes for the first four ingredients include using different vegetables or nuts based on personal preference. For example, kale can be used instead of broccoli in the salad, or almonds can be used instead of walnuts.

Tips include using a spiralizer to make zucchini noodles, or roasting the pine nuts before adding them to the pesto for extra flavor.

Radiant Roasted Vegetable Medley

Preparation Time: 30 minutes
Yield: 4 servings
Caloric Count: Approximately 150 calories per serving

Ingredients:
- 2 cups broccoli florets
- 1 cup cherry tomatoes
- 1 bell pepper, sliced
- 1 zucchini, sliced
- 2 tablespoons olive oil
- 1 teaspoon garlic powder
- Salt and pepper to taste

Method Of Preparation:
1. Preheat oven to 400°F (200°C).
2. Toss broccoli, cherry tomatoes, bell pepper, and zucchini with olive oil, garlic powder, salt, and pepper.
3. Roast in the oven for 20-25 minutes until golden.

Health Benefits:
- Broccoli contains indole-3-carbinol, aiding estrogen balance.
- Bell peppers provide vitamin C for collagen synthesis during menopause.

Substitutes:
- Use cauliflower instead of broccoli for variety.

Tips:
- Sprinkle in some nutritional yeast for a cheesy taste.

Savory Spinach Stuffed Mushrooms

Preparation Time: 25 minutes
Yield: 3 servings
Caloric Count: Approximately 120 calories per serving

Ingredients:
- 9 large mushrooms, cleaned and stems removed
- 2 cups spinach, chopped
- 1/2 cup feta cheese, crumbled
- 1 tablespoon olive oil
- 1 teaspoon balsamic vinegar
- Salt and pepper to taste

Method Of Preparation:
1. Preheat oven to 375°F (190°C).
2. In a pan, sauté spinach with olive oil until wilted. Mix in feta, balsamic vinegar, salt, and pepper.
3. Stuff mushrooms with the spinach mixture and bake for 15-20 minutes.

Health Benefits:
- Spinach provides iron, essential for energy during menopause.
- Feta contributes calcium for bone health.

Substitutes:
- Replace feta with goat cheese for a tangy twist.

Tips:
- Top with chopped walnuts for added crunch.

Cauliflower & Turmeric Mash

Preparation Time: 30 minutes
Yield: 4 servings
Caloric Count: Approximately 100 calories per serving

Ingredients:
- 1 head cauliflower, cut into florets
- 1 tablespoon coconut oil
- 1 teaspoon turmeric
- 1/2 teaspoon cumin
- Salt and pepper to taste
- Chopped chives for garnish

Method Of Preparation:
1. Steam cauliflower until tender.
2. Blend with coconut oil, turmeric, cumin, salt, and pepper until smooth.
3. Garnish with chopped chives.

Health Benefits:
- Turmeric has anti-inflammatory properties, beneficial for menopausal symptoms.
- Cauliflower is rich in phytonutrients supporting hormonal balance.

Substitutes:
- Swap coconut oil with olive oil.

Tips:
- Add a pinch of black pepper to enhance turmeric absorption.

Zesty Lemon Garlic Asparagus

Preparation Time: 20 minutes
Yield: 3 servings
Caloric Count: Approximately 80 calories per serving

Ingredients:
- 1 bunch asparagus, trimmed
- 2 tablespoons olive oil
- 2 cloves garlic, minced

- Zest of 1 lemon
- Salt and pepper to taste

Method Of Preparation:
1. Preheat oven to 425°F (220°C).
2. Toss asparagus with olive oil, minced garlic, lemon zest, salt, and pepper.
3. Roast for 12-15 minutes until tender-crisp.

Health Benefits:
- Asparagus is a source of folate, supporting cardiovascular health during menopause.
- Garlic contains allicin, known for its anti-inflammatory properties.

Substitutes:
- Use lime zest for a citrusy variation.

Tips:
- Sprinkle with crushed red pepper for a hint of spice.

Sweet Potato Kale Hash

Preparation Time: 30 minutes
Yield: 4 servings
Caloric Count: Approximately 180 calories per serving

Ingredients:
- 2 sweet potatoes, diced
- 2 cups kale, chopped
- 1 red onion, diced
- 2 tablespoons coconut oil
- 1 teaspoon smoked paprika
- Salt and pepper to taste

Method Of Preparation:
1. In a pan, sauté sweet potatoes, kale, and red onion in coconut oil until golden.
2. Season with smoked paprika, salt, and pepper.

Health Benefits:
- Sweet potatoes offer beta-carotene, vital for skin health.
- Kale contains calcium and vitamin K, supporting bone strength.

Substitutes:
- Replace coconut oil with avocado oil.

Tips:
- Top with a poached egg for added protein.

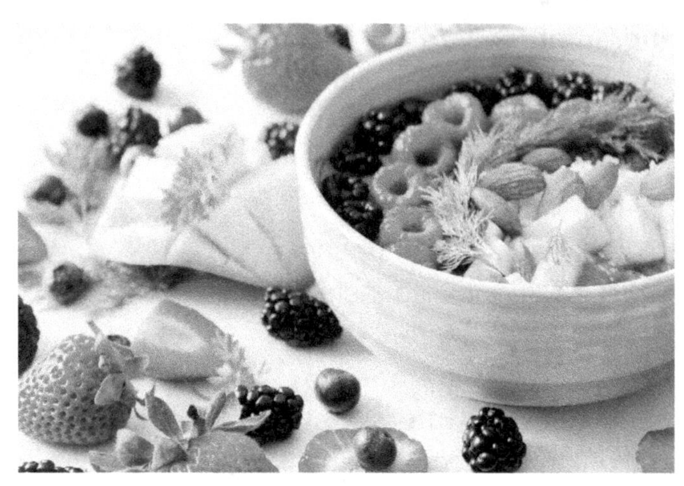

CHAPTER EIGHT

FISH/SEA FOOD RECIPES

Grilled Salmon Fillet with Asparagus

- **Preparation Time:** 20 minutes
- **Yield**: 4 servings
- **Caloric Count**: 400 calories per serving
- **Nutritional Information Per Serving:** 20g protein, 20g carb, 400mg sodium, 15g fat (3g sat), 7g fiber, 7g sugar (2g added sugar), 19g pro

- **Ingredients:**
  - 4 salmon fillets
  - 1 bunch asparagus
  - 1 tbsp olive oil
  - Salt and pepper to taste
  - 1 lemon, sliced

- **Method Of Preparation:**
  1. Warm the grill or grill pan to medium-high heat.
  2. Rinse and pat dry the salmon fillets with paper towels.
  3. Season the salmon fillets with salt and pepper.

4. Place the salmon fillets and asparagus on the grill or in the grill pan.

5. Top the salmon with lemon slices.

6. Grill for 5-7 minutes per side, or until the salmon is cooked through and the asparagus is tender.

7. Serve with a side salad or steamed vegetables for a complete meal.

Tequila Lime Shrimp Zoodles

- **Preparation Time:** 15 minutes
- **Yield**: 4 servings
- **Caloric Count**: 300 calories per serving
-**Nutritional Information Per Serving:** 12g protein, 20g carb, 200mg sodium, 10g fat (2g sat), 3g fiber, 7g sugar (2g added sugar), 15g pro

- **Ingredients**:
  - 1 lb large peeled and deveined shrimp
  - 2 tbsp olive oil
  - Salt and pepper to taste
  - 1 tbsp tequila
  - 1 tbsp lime juice
  - 1 garlic clove, minced
  - 1 tbsp honey
  - 1 tbsp chopped fresh cilantro
  - 4 zucchini, spiralized

- **Method Of Preparation:**

  1. Pat the shrimp dry and season with salt and pepper.

  2. Heat olive oil in a large nonstick skillet or wok over medium-high heat.

  3. Add the shrimp to the skillet and cook for 2-3 minutes per side, or until they turn pink.

  4. Remove the shrimp from the skillet and keep aside.

  5. In the same skillet, combine the tequila, lime juice, garlic, honey, and cilantro.

  6. Add the zucchini noodles to the skillet and cook for 2-3 minutes, stirring occasionally, until the noodles are tender.

  7. Return the shrimp to the skillet and cook for an additional 1-2 minutes, until heated through.

  8. Serve immediately.

Harissa Fish with Bulgur Salad

- **Preparation Time:** 20 minutes
- **Yield**: 4 servings
- **Caloric Count:** 450 calories per serving
- **Nutritional Information Per Serving:** 20g protein, 40g carb, 400mg sodium, 15g fat (3g sat), 5g fiber, 7g sugar (2g added sugar), 19g pro

- **Ingredients:**
  - 4 cod fillets

- 1 tbsp olive oil
- Salt and pepper to taste
- 2 tbsp harissa paste
- 1 cup cooked bulgur wheat
- 1/2 cup chopped fresh parsley
- 1/2 cup chopped fresh mint
- 1/4 cup chopped green onions
- 1/4 cup chopped cucumber
- 1/4 cup chopped cherry tomatoes
- 1/4 cup lemon juice
- 1 tbsp olive oil
- Salt and pepper to taste

- **Method Of Preparation**:

1. Pat the cod fillets dry and season with salt and pepper.

2. Heat olive oil in a large non-stick skillet or wok over medium-high heat.

3. Add the cod fillets to the skillet and cook for 2-3 minutes per side, or until they turn flaky and opaque.

4. Remove the cod fillets from the skillet and set aside.

5. In a large bowl, combine the bulgur wheat, parsley, mint, green onions, cucumber, cherry tomatoes, lemon juice, and olive oil.

6. Season the salad with salt and pepper to your taste.

7. Serve the grilled cod fillets over the bulgur salad.

Mediterranean Fish Gratin

- **Preparation Time:** 25 minutes
- **Yield**: 4 servings
- **Caloric Count**: 400 calories per serving
- **Nutritional Information Per Serving:** 20g protein, 40g carb, 400mg sodium, 15g fat (3g sat), 5g fiber, 7g sugar (2g added sugar), 19g protein

- **Ingredients**:
 - 4 cod fillets
 - 1 tbsp olive oil
 - Salt and pepper to taste
 - 1/2 cup chopped fresh parsley
 - 1/2 cup chopped fresh basil
 - 1/2 cup chopped fresh cherry tomatoes
 - 1/4 cup chopped green onions
 - 1/4 cup chopped cucumber
 - 1/4 cup lemon juice
 - 1 tbsp olive oil
 - Salt and pepper to taste
 - 1 cup grated mozzarella cheese

- **Method Of Preparation:**
 1. Pat the cod fillets dry and season with salt and pepper.

2. Heat olive oil in a large non stick skillet or wok over medium-high heat.

3. Add the cod fillets to the skillet and cook for 2-3 minutes per side, or until they turn flaky and opaque.

4. Remove the cod fillets from the skillet and set aside

Succulent Lemon Herb Salmon

Preparation Time: 25 minutes
Yield: 4 servings
Caloric Count: Approximately 250 calories per serving

Ingredients:
- 4 salmon fillets
- 2 tablespoons olive oil
- 1 lemon, sliced
- 2 teaspoons fresh dill, chopped
- 1 teaspoon garlic powder
- Salt and pepper to taste

Method of Preparation:
1. Preheat oven to 375°F (190°C).
2. Place salmon fillets on a baking sheet. Season with garlic powder, salt, pepper and drizzle with olive oil
3. Top with lemon slices and sprinkle with fresh dill. Bake for 15-20 minutes until flaky.

Health Benefits:
- Salmon is rich in omega-3 fatty acids, supporting heart health and hormonal balance during menopause.
- Dill contains phytoestrogens, aiding in estrogen regulation.

Substitutes:
- Substitute dill with parsley for a different herb flavor.

Tips:
- Serve over a bed of quinoa for a complete meal.

Zesty Shrimp and Avocado Salad

Preparation Time: 20 minutes
Yield: 3 servings
Caloric Count: Approximately 200 calories per serving

Ingredients:
- 300g shrimp, peeled and deveined
- 2 avocados, diced
- 1 cup cherry tomatoes, halved
- 2 tablespoons lime juice
- 1 tablespoon cilantro, chopped
- Salt and pepper to taste

Method of Preparation:
1. Sauté shrimp in a pan until cooked.
2. In a bowl, combine shrimp, diced avocados, cherry tomatoes, lime juice, cilantro, salt, and pepper.

Health Benefits:
- Shrimp provides iodine for thyroid health.
- Avocado offers monounsaturated fats, crucial for hormonal balance.

Substitutes:
- Use lemon juice if lime is not available.

Tips:
- Serve as a refreshing wrap using lettuce leaves.

Miso Glazed Cod with Sesame Broccoli

Preparation Time: 30 minutes
Yield: 2 servings
Caloric Count: Approximately 300 calories per serving

Ingredients:
- 2 cod fillets
- 2 tablespoons white miso paste

- 1 tablespoon honey
- 1 tablespoon soy sauce
- 1 teaspoon sesame oil
- 2 cups broccoli florets
- Sesame seeds for garnish

Method of Preparation:

1. Preheat oven to 400°F (200°C).
2. Mix miso paste, honey, soy sauce, and sesame oil. Brush over cod fillets.
3. Roast cod and broccoli in the oven for 15-20 minutes. Sprinkle with sesame seeds before serving.

Health Benefits:
- Cod is a lean source of protein, vital for muscle health.
- Miso paste contains probiotics, promoting gut health during menopause.

Substitutes:
- Use maple syrup instead of honey.

Tips:
- Garnish with sliced green onions for added freshness.

Spicy Garlic Butter Lobster Tails

Preparation Time: 35 minutes
Yield: 2 servings
Caloric Count: Approximately 280 calories per serving

Ingredients:
- 2 lobster tails
- 4 tablespoons butter, melted
- 3 cloves garlic, minced
- 1 teaspoon red pepper flakes
- 1 tablespoon fresh parsley, chopped
- Salt and pepper to taste

Method of Preparation:
1. Preheat oven to 425°F (220°C).
2. Butterfly lobster tails and place on a baking sheet.
3. Mix melted butter, minced garlic, red pepper flakes, salt, and pepper. Brush over lobster tails.
4. Bake for 15-20 minutes. Garnish with fresh parsley before serving.

Health Benefits:
- Lobster is rich in zinc, essential for immune function during menopause.
- Garlic contains allicin, known for its anti-inflammatory properties.

Substitutes:
- Use ghee instead of butter.

Tips:
- You can serve with a side of steamed vegetables for a well-balanced meal.

Coconut Lime Cilantro Grilled Fish Tacos

Preparation Time: 30 minutes
Yield: 6 tacos
Caloric Count: Approximately 220 calories per serving

Ingredients:
- 500g white fish fillets
- 2 tablespoons coconut oil, melted
- Zest and juice of 2 limes
- 2 tablespoons fresh cilantro, chopped
- 1 teaspoon cumin
- 6 small corn tortillas
- Shredded cabbage and sliced radishes for topping

Method of Preparation:
1. Marinate fish in coconut oil, lime zest, lime juice, cilantro, and cumin for 15 minutes.
2. Grill fish fillets until cooked through.

3. Assemble tacos with grilled fish, shredded cabbage, and sliced radishes on corn tortillas.

Health Benefits:
- White fish is a low-calorie, high-protein option for supporting muscle health.
- Coconut oil provides medium-chain triglycerides, promoting satiety during intermittent fasting.

Substitutes:
- For added fiber, use whole wheat tortillas.

Tips:
- Drizzle with extra lime juice for a burst of freshness.

CHAPTER NINE

POULTRY RECIPES

Turmeric Infused Grilled Chicken

Preparation Time: 30 minutes
Yield: 4 servings
Caloric Count: Approximately 280 calories per serving

Ingredients:
- 4 chicken breasts
- 2 tablespoons olive oil
- 1 teaspoon turmeric powder
- 1 teaspoon cumin
- 1 teaspoon smoked paprika
- Salt and pepper to taste

Method of Preparation:
1. In a bowl, mix olive oil, turmeric, cumin, smoked paprika, salt, and pepper.
2. Coat chicken breasts with the marinade and let sit for 15 minutes.
3. Grill chicken until fully cooked, about 6-8 minutes per side.

Health Benefits:

- Turmeric contains curcumin, known for its anti-inflammatory properties.
- Chicken is a lean protein source, crucial for muscle health during menopause.

Substitutes:
- Use boneless turkey breasts instead of chicken.

Tips:
- Serve with a side of colorful roasted vegetables for added nutrients.

Lemon Rosemary Baked Turkey Thighs

Preparation Time: 35 minutes
Yield: 3 servings
Caloric Count: Approximately 300 calories per serving

Ingredients:
- 3 turkey thighs
- 2 tablespoons melted ghee
- Zest and juice of 1 lemon
- 2 teaspoons fresh rosemary, chopped
- 3 cloves garlic, minced
- Salt and pepper to taste

Method of Preparation:
1. Preheat oven to 400°F (200°C).
2. Mix melted ghee, lemon zest, lemon juice, rosemary, minced garlic, salt, and pepper.
3. Coat turkey thighs with the mixture and bake for 25-30 minutes.

Health Benefits:
- Turkey is rich in tryptophan, promoting serotonin production for mood regulation.
- Rosemary contains antioxidants linked to improved cognitive function.

Substitutes:
- Substitute ghee with olive oil.

Tips:
- Serve with a quinoa salad for a complete meal.

Mango Chili Lime Chicken Skewers

Preparation Time: 25 minutes
Yield: 4 servings
Caloric Count: Approximately 250 calories per serving

Ingredients:
- 1.5 lbs boneless, skinless chicken thighs, cut into chunks

- 1 mango, peeled and diced
- 2 tablespoons olive oil
- Zest and juice of 2 limes
- 1 teaspoon chili powder
- Salt and pepper to taste

Method of Preparation:

1. In a blender, puree mango, olive oil, lime zest, lime juice, chili powder, salt, and pepper.
2. Thread chicken chunks onto skewers and brush with the mango mixture.
3. Grill skewers for 10-12 minutes, turning occasionally.

Health Benefits:

- Mango provides vitamin E, supporting skin health during menopause.
- Chili powder contains capsaicin, known for its metabolism-boosting properties.

Substitutes:

- Use chicken breasts instead of thighs.

Tips:

- Serve over a bed of cauliflower rice for a low-carb option.

Spinach and Feta Stuffed Chicken Breast

Preparation Time: 40 minutes
Yield: 2 servings
Caloric Count: Approximately 320 calories per serving

Ingredients:
- 2 boneless, skinless chicken breasts
- 2 cups fresh spinach, chopped
- 1/2 cup feta cheese, crumbled
- 2 tablespoons olive oil
- 1 teaspoon garlic powder
- Salt and pepper to taste

Method of Preparation:
1. Preheat oven to 375°F (190°C).
2. Butterfly chicken breasts and season with garlic powder, salt, and pepper.
3. Mix chopped spinach and feta. Stuff each chicken breast with the mixture and secure with toothpicks.
4. In a pan, heat olive oil. Sear chicken for 2 minutes on each side. Transfer to the oven and bake for 20-25 minutes.

Health Benefits:
- Spinach is rich in iron, supporting energy levels during menopause.

- Feta provides calcium for bone health.

Substitutes:
- Use goat cheese instead of feta.

Tips:
- Drizzle with balsamic reduction for added flavor.

Crispy Garlic Parmesan Chicken Tenders

Preparation Time: 30 minutes
Yield: 4 servings
Caloric Count: Approximately 260 calories per serving

Ingredients:
- 1.5 lbs chicken tenders
- 1 cup almond flour
- 1/2 cup grated Parmesan cheese
- 2 teaspoons garlic powder
- 2 eggs, beaten
- Salt and pepper to taste

Method of Preparation:
1. Preheat oven to 400°F (200°C).
2. Mix almond flour, Parmesan, garlic powder, salt, and pepper in a bowl.

3. Dip chicken tenders in beaten eggs, then coat with the almond flour mixture.

4. Bake for over 20-25 minutes until golden and crispy.

Health Benefits:

- Almond flour is a low-carb alternative, suitable for those watching their carbohydrate intake.

- Parmesan cheese offers protein and calcium.

Substitutes:

- You can opt for coconut flour instead of almond flour.

Tips:

- Serve with a side of homemade tomato sauce for dipping.

Balsamic Glazed Rosemary Chicken

Preparation Time: 35 minutes
Yield: 3 servings
Caloric Count: Approximately 290 calories per serving

Ingredients:
- 3 chicken thighs, bone-in, skin-on
- 3 tablespoons balsamic vinegar
- 2 tablespoons honey

- 1 tablespoon fresh rosemary, chopped
- 2 cloves garlic, minced
- Salt and pepper to taste

Method of Preparation:
1. Preheat oven to 375°F (190°C).
2. Mix balsamic vinegar, honey, chopped rosemary, minced garlic, salt, and pepper.
3. Coat chicken thighs with the mixture and bake for 25-30 minutes.

Health Benefits:
- Balsamic vinegar contains antioxidants linked to heart health.
- Rosemary may have neuroprotective properties, beneficial during menopause.

Substitutes:
- Use maple syrup instead of honey.

Tips:
- Serve with a side of quinoa and roasted vegetables.

Sesame Ginger Glazed Chicken Stir-Fry

Preparation Time: 30 minutes
Yield: 4 servings

Caloric Count: Approximately 260 calories per serving

Ingredients:
- 1.5 lbs chicken breast, thinly sliced
- 3 tablespoons soy sauce
- 2 tablespoons sesame oil
- 1 tablespoon fresh ginger, grated
- 2 cloves garlic, minced
- 1 tablespoon honey
- 2 cups broccoli florets
- 1 bell pepper, sliced
- 2 green onions, sliced

Method of Preparation:
1. In a bowl, mix soy sauce, sesame oil, grated ginger, minced garlic, and honey.
2. Stir-fry chicken in a pan until cooked, then add broccoli and bell pepper.
3. Pour the sauce over the stir-fry, cooking until the vegetables are tender.
4. Garnish with sliced green onions.

Health Benefits:
- Ginger has anti-inflammatory properties, aiding in menopausal symptom relief.
- Broccoli provides fiber for digestive health.

Substitutes:

- Opt for tamari instead of soy sauce for a gluten-free option.

Tips:

- Serve over cauliflower rice for a low-carb twist.

Pomegranate Glazed Chicken Salad

Preparation Time: 25 minutes
Yield: 3 servings
Caloric Count: Approximately 280 calories per serving

Ingredients:
- 3 chicken breasts
- 1/2 cup pomegranate juice
- 2 tablespoons olive oil
- 1 tablespoon Dijon mustard
- 1 tablespoon honey
- Mixed salad greens
- 1/4 cup pomegranate seeds

Method of Preparation:
1. Grill chicken until fully cooked.
2. In a bowl, whisk together pomegranate juice, olive oil, Dijon mustard, and honey.

3. Slice chicken and arrange on a bed of mixed salad greens. Drizzle with the pomegranate dressing and sprinkle with pomegranate seeds.

Health Benefits:
- Pomegranate juice is rich in antioxidants, supporting heart health.
- Dijon mustard adds flavor without excess calories.

Substitutes:
- Instead of honey, use maple
 in the dressing.

Tips:
- Top with toasted walnuts for added crunch.

Mediterranean Chicken Skillet

Preparation Time: 35 minutes
Yield: 4 servings
Caloric Count: Approximately 310 calories per serving

Ingredients:
- 4 chicken thighs, bone-in, skin-on
- 2 tablespoons olive oil
- 1 onion, sliced
- 2 bell peppers, sliced
- 3 cloves garlic, minced

- 1 teaspoon dried oregano
- 1 teaspoon smoked paprika
- 1/2 cup cherry tomatoes, halved
- Feta cheese for garnish

Method of Preparation:

1. Season chicken thighs with salt, pepper, oregano, and smoked paprika.
2. In a skillet, heat olive oil and sear chicken until golden. Remove from skillet.
3. In the same skillet, sauté onions, bell peppers, and garlic until softened. Add cherry tomatoes and return chicken to the skillet.
4. Bake in the oven at 375°F (190°C) for 20-25 minutes.
5. Garnish with crumbled feta before serving.

Health Benefits:

- Olive oil provides monounsaturated fats, supporting heart health.
- Bell peppers offer vitamin C, crucial for collagen production.

Substitutes:

- Use boneless, skinless chicken breasts for a lighter option.

Tips:

- Serve over quinoa or brown rice.

Cajun Spiced Chicken Lettuce Wraps

Preparation Time: 20 minutes
Yield: 4 servings
Caloric Count: Approximately 240 calories per serving

Ingredients:
- 1.5 lbs chicken breast, diced
- 2 tablespoons Cajun seasoning
- 1 tablespoon olive oil
- 1 avocado, sliced
- 1 cup cherry tomatoes, halved
- 1/2 cup Greek yogurt
- Lettuce leaves for wrapping

Method of Preparation:
1. Toss diced chicken with Cajun seasoning.
2. In a pan, heat olive oil and cook the seasoned chicken until done.
3. Assemble lettuce wraps with chicken, avocado slices, and cherry tomatoes. Top with Greek yogurt.

Health Benefits:
- Avocado gives healthy fats for hormone production.
- Greek yogurt offers probiotics for gut health.

Substitutes:
- You can alternate with sour cream instead of Greek yogurt.

CHAPTER TEN

MEAT RECIPES

Ginger Garlic Glazed Beef Stir-Fry

Preparation Time: 30 minutes
Yield: 4 servings
Caloric Count: Approximately 320 calories per serving

Ingredients:
1.5 lbs beef sirloin, thinly sliced
3 tablespoons soy sauce
2 tablespoons sesame oil
1 tablespoon fresh ginger, grated
2 cloves garlic, minced
1 tablespoon honey
2 cups broccoli florets
1 bell pepper, sliced
2 green onions, sliced

Method of Preparation:
In a bowl, mix soy sauce, sesame oil, grated ginger, minced garlic, and honey.
Stir-fry beef until cooked, then add broccoli and bell pepper.
Pour the sauce over the stir-fry, cooking until the vegetables are tender.

Garnish with sliced green onions.

Health Benefits:
Ginger has anti-inflammatory properties, aiding in menopausal symptom relief.
Broccoli provides fiber for digestive health.

Substitutes:
Oot for tamari instead of soy sauce for a gluten-free option.

Tips:
Serve over cauliflower rice for a low-carb twist.
 Mango Chili Lime Pork Chops
Preparation Time: 25 minutes
Yield: 3 servings
Caloric Count: Approximately 280 calories per serving

Ingredients:
3 pork chops
1 mango, peeled and diced
2 tablespoons olive oil
Zest and juice of 2 limes
1 teaspoon chili powder
Salt and pepper to taste

Method of Preparation:
In a blender, puree mango, olive oil, lime zest, lime juice, chili powder, salt, and pepper.
Season pork chops with the mango mixture and let marinate for 15 minutes.
Grill pork chops until fully cooked.

Health Benefits:
Mango provides vitamin E, supporting skin health during menopause.
Chili powder contains capsaicin, known for its metabolism-boosting properties.

Substitutes:
Use boneless chicken thighs instead of pork.

Tips:
Serve with a side of quinoa or brown rice.

Lemon Herb Turkey Skillet

Preparation Time: 30 minutes
Yield: 4 servings
Caloric Count: Approximately 300 calories per serving

Ingredients:
1.5 lbs ground turkey
2 tablespoons olive oil
Zest and juice of 1 lemon

2 teaspoons fresh thyme, chopped
2 cloves garlic, minced
1 teaspoon onion powder
Salt and pepper to taste
1 cup cherry tomatoes, halved

Method of Preparation:
In a skillet, brown ground turkey in olive oil.
Add lemon zest, lemon juice, chopped thyme, minced garlic, onion powder, salt, and pepper.
Stir in cherry tomatoes and cook until heated through.
Health Benefits:
Turkey is a lean source of protein, crucial for muscle health during menopause.
Lemon provides vitamin C, supporting collagen production.

Substitutes:
Use ground chicken if turkey is not available.

Tips:
Serve over a bed of spinach for added nutrients.

Cumin Spiced Lamb Kebabs

Preparation Time: 35 minutes
Yield: 3 servings

Caloric Count: Approximately 330 calories per serving

Ingredients:
1.5 lbs lamb, cubed
2 tablespoons Greek yogurt
1 tablespoon ground cumin
1 teaspoon smoked paprika
2 cloves garlic, minced
2 tablespoons olive oil
Salt and pepper to taste

Method of Preparation:
In a bowl, mix Greek yogurt, ground cumin, smoked paprika, minced garlic, olive oil, salt, and pepper.
Marinate lamb cubes in the mixture for 20 minutes.
Thread lamb onto skewers and grill until cooked.

Health Benefits:
Lamb is a good source of heme iron, supporting energy levels during menopause.
Greek yogurt provides probiotics for gut health.

Substitutes:
Use beef cubes if lamb is not preferred.

Tips:
Serve with a side of tzatziki sauce.

Cherry Balsamic Glazed Chicken
Preparation Time: 40 minutes
Yield: 4 servings
Caloric Count: Approximately 310 calories per serving

Ingredients:
4 chicken breasts
1 cup cherries, pitted and halved
3 tablespoons balsamic vinegar
2 tablespoons olive oil
1 tablespoon honey
1 teaspoon rosemary, chopped
Salt and pepper to taste

Method of Preparation:
Preheat oven to 375°F (190°C).
In a saucepan, combine cherries, balsamic vinegar, olive oil, honey, chopped rosemary, salt, and pepper. Simmer until cherries soften.
Season chicken breasts and bake in the oven for 25-30 minutes.
Spoon the cherry balsamic glaze over the cooked chicken before serving.

Health Benefits:
Cherries contain melatonin, aiding in sleep regulation during menopause.
Blood sugar regulation may be assisted by using balsamic vinegar.

Substitutes:
For the glaze, use maple syrup in place of the honey.

Tips:
Garnish with fresh mint for a burst of freshness.

Mushroom and Spinach Stuffed Pork Tenderloin

Preparation Time: 35 minutes
Yield: 3 servings
Caloric Count: Approximately 290 calories per serving

Ingredients:
1 pork tenderloin
2 cups baby spinach, chopped
1 cup mushrooms, finely chopped
3 tablespoons goat cheese, crumbled
2 tablespoons olive oil
1 teaspoon dried thyme
Salt and pepper to taste

Method of Preparation:
Preheat oven to 400°F (200°C).
Butterfly the pork tenderloin.
In a pan, sauté chopped spinach, mushrooms, and goat cheese in olive oil until wilted. Add dried thyme, salt, and pepper.
Spread the spinach-mushroom mixture on the butterflied pork and roll it up. Secure with toothpicks.
Roast in the oven for 25-30 minutes.

Health Benefits:
Spinach provides iron, crucial for energy during menopause.
Goat cheese offers a dose of calcium for bone health.

Substitutes:
Use feta instead of goat cheese.

Tips:
Drizzle with balsamic reduction for added flavor.

Orange Glazed Teriyaki Chicken

Preparation Time: 30 minutes
Yield: 4 servings

Caloric Count: Approximately 280 calories per serving

Ingredients:
4 chicken thighs, bone-in, skin-on
1/2 cup teriyaki sauce
Zest and juice of 1 orange
2 tablespoons honey
1 tablespoon sesame seeds
1 teaspoon ginger, grated
2 tablespoons green onions, sliced

Method of Preparation:
Preheat oven to 375°F (190°C).
In a bowl, mix teriyaki sauce, orange zest, orange juice, honey, sesame seeds, and grated ginger.
Coat chicken thighs with the mixture and bake for 25-30 minutes.
Garnish with sliced green onions before serving.

Health Benefits:
Oranges provide vitamin C, supporting immune health.
Teriyaki sauce offers a savory flavor without excessive sodium.

Substitutes:
Use tamari for a gluten-free teriyaki alternative.

Tips:
Serve over a bed of brown rice.

Sesame Ginger Glazed Salmon

Preparation Time: 25 minutes
Yield: 3 servings
Caloric Count: Approximately 260 calories per serving

Ingredients:
3 salmon fillets
3 tablespoons soy sauce
2 tablespoons honey
1 tablespoon sesame oil
1 teaspoon fresh ginger, grated
1 clove garlic, minced
Sesame seeds for garnish
Green onions for garnish

Method of Preparation:
Preheat oven to 400°F (200°C).
In a bowl, mix soy sauce, honey, sesame oil, grated ginger, and minced garlic.
Brush the mixture over salmon fillets and bake for 15-20 minutes.
Garnish with sesame seeds and sliced green onions before serving.

Health Benefits:
Salmon is rich in omega-3 fatty acids, supporting heart health and hormonal balance. Ginger has anti-inflammatory properties, beneficial during menopause.

Substitutes:
Use maple syrup instead of honey.

Tips:
Serve with steamed broccoli for added nutrients.

Tomato Basil Turkey Meatballs

Preparation Time: 30 minutes
Yield: 4 servings
Caloric Count: Approximately 280 calories per serving

Ingredients:
1.5 lbs ground turkey
1 cup breadcrumbs
1/2 cup Parmesan cheese, grated
1/4 cup fresh basil, chopped
1 egg
2 cloves garlic, minced
1 can (14 oz) crushed tomatoes
1 teaspoon dried oregano
Salt and pepper to taste

Method of Preparation:
Preheat oven to 375°F (190°C).
In a bowl, mix ground turkey, breadcrumbs, grated Parmesan, chopped basil, egg, minced garlic, salt, and pepper.
Place the formed meatballs on a baking sheet.
In a saucepan, heat crushed tomatoes, dried oregano, salt, and pepper. Simmer for 10 minutes.
Bake meatballs in the oven for 20-25 minutes.
Serve with tomato sauce.

Health Benefits:
Turkey is a lean protein source, crucial for muscle health during menopause.
Basil provides antioxidants, supporting overall health.

Substitutes:
Use ground chicken instead of turkey.

Tips:
Serve over zucchini noodles for a low-carb option.

Bacon-Wrapped Asparagus Stuffed Chicken

Preparation Time: 35 minutes
Yield: 3 servings
Caloric Count: Approximately 330 calories per serving

Ingredients:
3 chicken breasts
9 asparagus spears
3 slices bacon
1 tablespoon olive oil
1 teaspoon garlic powder
Salt and pepper to taste

Method of Preparation:
Preheat oven to 375°F (190°C).
Season the chicken breasts
to taste with salt, pepper and garlic powder.
Place 3 asparagus spears on each chicken breast and wrap with a slice of bacon.
In a pan, heat olive oil. Sear the bacon-wrapped chicken until bacon is crispy.
Transfer to the oven and bake for 20-25 minutes.

Health Benefits:
Asparagus is a good source of folate, important during menopause.

Olive oil provides monounsaturated fats, supporting heart health.

Substitutes:
Use turkey bacon for a leaner option.

Tips:
Drizzle with balsamic reduction for added flavor.

Citrus-Infused Grilled Chicken

Preparation Time: 30 minutes
Yield: 4 servings
Caloric Count: Approximately 270 calories per serving

Ingredients:
4 boneless, skinless chicken breasts
Zest and juice of 2 oranges
2 tablespoons olive oil
1 tablespoon honey
1 teaspoon thyme, chopped
Salt and pepper to taste

Method of Preparation:
In a bowl, mix orange zest, orange juice, olive oil, honey, chopped thyme, salt, and pepper.

Marinate chicken breasts in the mixture for 15 minutes.
Grill until fully cooked, about 6-8 minutes per side.

Health Benefits:
Oranges provide vitamin C, essential for collagen synthesis.
Thyme contains phytoestrogens, contributing to hormonal balance.

Substitutes:
Use lime instead of orange for a different citrus flavor.

Tips:
Serve with a side of quinoa and steamed broccoli for a balanced meal.

Sesame Ginger Turkey Meatballs

Preparation Time: 35 minutes
Yield: 3 servings
Caloric Count: Approximately 290 calories per serving

Ingredients:
1 lb ground turkey
2 tablespoons soy sauce
1 tablespoon sesame oil

1 tablespoon fresh ginger, grated
2 cloves garlic, minced
2 green onions, finely chopped
1/4 cup breadcrumbs (or preferably, almond flour for a gluten-free option)

Method of Preparation:
Preheat oven to 375°F (190°C).
In a bowl, mix ground turkey, soy sauce, sesame oil, grated ginger, minced garlic, green onions, and breadcrumbs.
Form into meatballs and bake for 20-25 minutes.

Health Benefits:
Turkey is a lean protein source, crucial for muscle health.
Ginger has anti-inflammatory properties, beneficial during menopause.

Substitutes:
You can opt for tamari instead of soy sauce for a gluten-free option.

Tips:
Serve with a side of cauliflower rice and sautéed spinach.

Mediterranean Lamb Skewers

Preparation Time: 30 minutes
Yield: 4 servings
Caloric Count: Approximately 320 calories per serving

Ingredients:
1.5 lbs lamb cubes
2 tablespoons olive oil
1 tablespoon lemon juice
1 teaspoon cumin
1 teaspoon paprika
2 cloves garlic, minced
Salt and pepper to taste

Method of Preparation:
In a bowl, mix olive oil, lemon juice, cumin, paprika, minced garlic, salt, and pepper.
Marinate lamb cubes in the mixture for 15 minutes.
Thread onto skewers and grill for 10-12 minutes.

Health Benefits:
Lamb is a good source of iron, supporting energy levels during menopause.
Cumin contains phytoestrogens, contributing to hormonal balance.

Substitutes:
Use ground coriander instead of cumin for a different flavor.

Tips:
Serve with a side of Greek salad.

Chili Lime Beef Stir-Fry

Preparation Time: 25 minutes
Yield: 3 servings
Caloric Count: Approximately 300 calories per serving

Ingredients:
1 lb beef sirloin, thinly sliced
3 tablespoons soy sauce
Zest and juice of 2 limes
1 tablespoon chili powder
2 tablespoons olive oil
1 bell pepper, sliced
1 cup snap peas
2 cloves garlic, minced

Method of Preparation:
In a bowl, mix soy sauce, lime zest, lime juice, and chili powder.
In a wok or skillet, heat olive oil and stir-fry beef until browned. Add minced garlic.

Add bell pepper and snap peas, then pour the sauce over. Stir-fry until vegetables are tender.

Health Benefits:

Beef provides iron, crucial for maintaining energy levels.

Chili powder contains capsaicin, known for its metabolism-boosting properties.

Substitutes:

You can opt for tamari instead of soy sauce for a gluten-free option.

Tips:

For a low-carb option, serve over cauliflower rice.

Coconut Lime Chicken Curry

Preparation Time: 40 minutes
Yield: 4 servings
Caloric Count: Approximately 340 calories per serving

Ingredients:

1.5 lbs chicken thighs, bone-in, skin-on
2 tablespoons coconut oil
1 onion, finely chopped
2 tablespoons red curry paste
1 can (14 oz) coconut milk
Zest and juice of 2 limes

1 tablespoon fish sauce
1 tablespoon cilantro, chopped

Method of Preparation:
In a pot, heat coconut oil and sauté onions until soft.
Add red curry paste and cook for 1-2 minutes.
Add chicken thighs, coconut milk, lime zest, lime juice, and fish sauce. Simmer until chicken is cooked through.
Garnish with chopped cilantro before serving.

Health Benefits:
Coconut milk provides healthy fats beneficial for hormonal balance.
Limes offer vitamin C, supporting immune health.

Substitutes:
Use chicken breasts instead of thighs.

Tips:
 Serve alongside cauliflower rice for a low-carb choice.

CHAPTER ELEVEN

SNACK RECIPES

Dark Chocolate Avocado Mousse

Preparation Time: 15 minutes
Yield: 2 servings
Caloric Count: Approximately 200 calories per serving

Ingredients:
- 2 ripe avocados
- 1/4 cup unsweetened cocoa powder
- 1/4 cup maple syrup
- 1 teaspoon vanilla extract
- A pinch of sea salt

Method of Preparation:
1. In a blender, combine avocados, cocoa powder, maple syrup, vanilla extract, and sea salt.
2. Blend until smooth and creamy.
3. Keep it refrigerated for at least 30 minutes before serving.

Health Benefits:
- Avocados are rich in monounsaturated fats, supporting hormone production.

- Dark chocolate contains antioxidants that may benefit heart health.

Substitutes:
- Use honey instead of maple syrup.

Tips:
- Garnish with a sprinkle of chopped nuts for added crunch.

Turmeric Almond Energy Bites

Preparation Time: 20 minutes
Yield: 12 bites
Caloric Count: Approximately 80 calories per bite

Ingredients:
- 1 cup rolled oats
- 1/2 cup almond butter
- 1/4 cup honey
- 1 teaspoon ground turmeric
- 1/2 teaspoon cinnamon
- 1/4 cup chia seeds

Method of Preparation:
1. In a bowl, mix rolled oats, almond butter, honey, ground turmeric, cinnamon, and chia seeds.

2. Form into bite-sized balls and refrigerate for at least 15 minutes.

Health Benefits:
- Turmeric has anti-inflammatory properties that may alleviate menopausal symptoms.
- Almond butter provides healthy fats for hormonal balance.

Substitutes:
- Use peanut butter instead of almond butter.

Tips:
- Roll the bites in shredded coconut for extra flavor.

Greek Yogurt Berry Parfait

Preparation Time: 10 minutes
Yield: 2 servings
Caloric Count: Approximately 150 calories per serving

Ingredients:
- 1 cup Greek yogurt
- 1/2 cup mixed berries (blueberries, strawberries, raspberries)
- 2 tablespoons honey

- 2 tablespoons chopped nuts (almonds, walnuts)

Method of Preparation:
1. In a glass, layer Greek yogurt, mixed berries, and drizzle with honey.
2. Repeat the layers.
3. Top with chopped nuts before serving.

Health Benefits:
- Greek yogurt provides probiotics for gut health.
- Berries offer antioxidants that support overall well-being.

Substitutes:
- Use maple syrup instead of honey.

Tips:
- Add a sprinkle of cinnamon for extra flavor.

Chickpea and Roasted Red Pepper Hummus

Preparation Time: 20 minutes
Yield: 2 cups
Caloric Count: Approximately 50 calories per tablespoon

Ingredients:

- 1 can (15 oz) of drained and rinsed chickpeas,
- 1/2 cup roasted red peppers
- 1/4 cup tahini
- 2 tablespoons olive oil
- 2 cloves garlic, minced
- Juice of 1 lemon
- Salt and pepper to taste

Method of Preparation:
1. In a food processor, blend chickpeas, roasted red peppers, tahini, olive oil, minced garlic, and lemon juice until smooth.
2. Season with salt and pepper.
3. Serve with vegetable sticks or whole-grain crackers.

Health Benefits:
- Chickpeas provide fiber, aiding in digestive health.
- Olive oil offers monounsaturated fats, beneficial for hormonal balance.

Substitutes:
- Use canned green peas instead of chickpeas.

Tips:
- Garnish with a drizzle of extra virgin olive oil.

Walnut and Date Protein Bars

Preparation Time: 25 minutes
Yield: 8 bars
Caloric Count: Approximately 180 calories per bar

Ingredients:
- 1 cup walnuts
- 1 cup pitted dates
- 1/4 cup protein powder (plant-based or whey)
- 1/4 cup unsweetened shredded coconut
- 1 teaspoon vanilla extract
- A pinch of sea salt

Method of Preparation:
1. In a food processor, blend walnuts, dates, protein powder, shredded coconut, vanilla extract, and sea salt until a sticky dough forms.
2. Press the mixture into a lined pan and refrigerate for 1 hour.
3. Cut into bars before serving.

Health Benefits:
- Walnuts contain omega-3 fatty acids, supporting heart health.
- Dates provide natural sweetness without added sugars.

Substitutes:
- Use almonds instead of walnuts.

Tips:
- Drizzle with melted dark chocolate for a decadent touch.

Edamame and Avocado Dip

Preparation Time: 15 minutes
Yield: 1 cup
Caloric Count: Approximately 120 calories per 1/4 cup

Ingredients:
- 1 cup shelled edamame, cooked
- 1 ripe avocado
- 1 tablespoon lime juice
- 1 tablespoon olive oil
- 1 clove garlic, minced
- Salt and pepper to taste

Method of Preparation:
1. In a blender, combine edamame, avocado, lime juice, olive oil, minced garlic, salt, and pepper.
2. Blend until smooth.
3. Serve with vegetable sticks or whole-grain crackers.

Health Benefits:
- Edamame is a soy-based protein source with potential benefits for menopausal symptoms.
- Avocado provides healthy monounsaturated fats.

Substitutes:
- Use lemon juice instead of lime.

Tips:
- A dash of cayenne pepper can be added for extra heat.

Cucumber and Salmon Roll-Ups

Preparation Time: 15 minutes
Yield: 2 servings
Caloric Count: Approximately 120 calories per serving

Ingredients:
- 1 cucumber, peeled into strips
- 4 oz smoked salmon
- 1/4 cup cream cheese
- 2 tablespoons capers
- Fresh dill for garnish

Method of Preparation:

1. Lay cucumber strips flat and spread a thin layer of cream cheese.
2. Place smoked salmon over the cream cheese.
3. Sprinkle with capers and roll up each strip.
4. Secure with toothpicks and garnish with fresh dill.

Health Benefits:
- Salmon provides omega-3 fatty acids, supporting heart and brain health.
- Cucumbers offer hydration and are low in calories.

Substitutes:
- Greek yogurt can be substituted for cream cheese.

Tips:
- Squeeze a bit of lemon juice for added freshness.

Black bean and Quinoa Stuffed Bell Peppers

Preparation Time: 30 minutes
Yield: 4 servings
Caloric Count: Approximately 180 calories per serving

Ingredients:
- 2 bell peppers, halved and deseeded
- 1/2 cup cooked quinoa
- 1/2 cup black beans, drained and rinsed
- 1/4 cup salsa
- 1/4 cup shredded cheese
- 1 teaspoon cumin
- 1/2 teaspoon chili powder

Method of Preparation:
1. Preheat oven to 375°F (190°C).
2. In a bowl, mix quinoa, black beans, salsa, shredded cheese, cumin, and chili powder.
3. Stuff each bell pepper half with the quinoa mixture.
4. Bake for over 20-25 minutes until peppers are soft

Health Benefits:
- Quinoa is a complete protein, essential for muscle health.
- Black beans provide fiber for digestive health.

Substitutes:
- Use brown rice instead of quinoa.

Tips:
- Top with sliced avocado before serving.

Kale and Sweet Potato Chips

Preparation Time: 30 minutes
Yield: 4 servings
Caloric Count: Approximately 100 calories per serving

Ingredients:
- 1 bunch kale, stems removed and torn into pieces
- 1 sweet potato, thinly sliced
- 2 tablespoons olive oil
- 1 teaspoon paprika
- 1/2 teaspoon garlic powder
- Salt and pepper to taste

Method of Preparation:
1. Preheat oven to 375°F (190°C).
2. Toss kale and sweet potato slices with olive oil, paprika, garlic powder, salt, and pepper.
3. Spread on baking sheets and bake for 15-20 minutes until crispy.

Health Benefits:
- Kale is rich in calcium and vitamin K, supporting bone health.
- Sweet potatoes provide beta-carotene, essential for skin health.

Substitutes:

- You can use coconut oil as an alternative instead of olive oil.

Tips:
- Sprinkle nutritional yeast for an extra cheesy flavor.

Protein-Packed Cottage Cheese with Berries

Preparation Time: 10 minutes
Yield: 2 servings
Caloric Count: Approximately 150 calories per serving

Ingredients:
- 1 cup low-fat cottage cheese
- 1/2 cup mixed berries (strawberries, blueberries, raspberries)
- 1 tablespoon honey
- 2 tablespoons chopped nuts (almonds, walnuts)

Method of Preparation:
1. In a bowl, spoon cottage cheese.
2. Top with mixed berries.
3. Drizzle with honey and sprinkle chopped nuts.

Health Benefits:

- Cottage cheese is high in protein, essential for muscle health.
- Berries provide antioxidants that support overall well-being.

Substitutes:
- Use Greek yogurt instead of cottage cheese.

Tips:
- Add a dash of cinnamon for extra flavor.

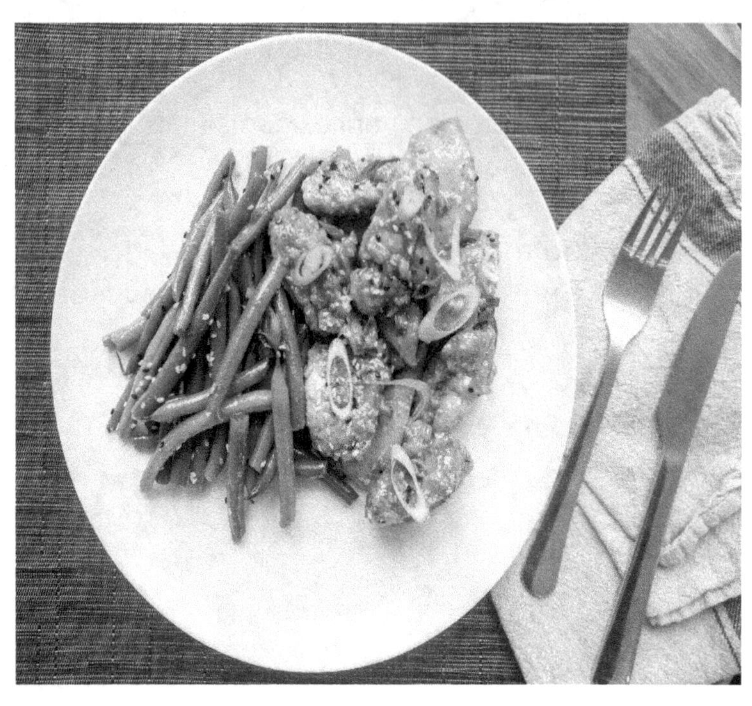

CHAPTER TWELVE

DESSERTS RECIPES

Cocoa-Dusted Almond Butter Banana Bites

Preparation Time: 15 minutes
Yield: 4 servings
Caloric Count: Approximately 130 calories per serving

Ingredients:
- 2 bananas, sliced
- 1/4 cup almond butter
- 2 tablespoons unsweetened cocoa powder
- 1 tablespoon honey
- Crushed almonds for garnish

Method of Preparation:
1. Spread almond butter on banana slices.
2. In a shallow dish, mix cocoa powder and honey.
3. Dip each banana slice into the cocoa mixture to coat.
4. Garnish with crushed almonds.

Health Benefits:

- Bananas provide potassium, which are crucial for heart health.
- Almond butter offers healthy fats and protein.

Substitutes:
- Use peanut butter instead of almond butter.

Tips:
- Chill in the refrigerator for a firmer texture.

Pomegranate and Greek Yogurt Parfait

Preparation Time: 10 minutes
Yield: 2 servings
Caloric Count: Approximately 160 calories per serving

Ingredients:
- 1 cup Greek yogurt
- 1/2 cup pomegranate seeds
- 2 tablespoons honey
- 2 tablespoons granola

Method of Preparation:
1. In a glass, layer Greek yogurt, pomegranate seeds, and granola.
2. Repeat the layers.
3. Drizzle with honey before serving.

Health Benefits:
- Pomegranate seeds are rich in antioxidants that may support heart health.
- Greek yogurt provides probiotics for gut health.

Substitutes:
- Use maple syrup instead of honey.

Tips:
- Top with a sprinkle of flaxseeds for added fiber.

Almond Flour Blueberry Muffins

Preparation Time: 25 minutes
Yield: 8 muffins
Caloric Count: Approximately 150 calories per muffin

Ingredients:
- 2 cups almond flour
- 1/4 cup coconut flour
- 1/4 cup honey
- 1/4 cup coconut oil, melted
- 3 large eggs
- 1 teaspoon vanilla extract
- 1/2 teaspoon baking soda
- 1/4 teaspoon salt
- 1 cup blueberries

Method of Preparation:

1. Preheat oven to 350°F (175°C) and line a muffin tin with paper liners.
2. In a bowl, mix almond flour, coconut flour, honey, melted coconut oil, eggs, vanilla extract, baking soda, and salt.
3. Gently fold in blueberries.
4. Divide the batter into muffin cups and bake for 20-22 minutes.

Health Benefits:

- Almond flour is a low-carb alternative, supporting stable blood sugar levels.
- Blueberries are rich in antioxidants that may benefit cognitive function.

Substitutes:

- Use ghee instead of coconut oil.

Tips:

- Sprinkle with sliced almonds for added crunch.

Coconut and Matcha Green Tea Energy Bites

Preparation Time: 20 minutes
Yield: 12 bites

Caloric Count: Approximately 90 calories per bite

Ingredients:
- 1 cup shredded coconut
- 1/2 cup almond flour
- 1/4 cup coconut oil, melted
- 2 tablespoons honey
- 1 teaspoon matcha green tea powder
- 1/2 teaspoon vanilla extract

Method of Preparation:
1. In a bowl, combine shredded coconut, almond flour, melted coconut oil, honey, matcha green tea powder, and vanilla extract.
2. Form into bite-sized balls and refrigerate for 1 hour.

Health Benefits:
- Matcha green tea contains antioxidants and may support metabolism.
- Coconut oil provides medium-chain triglycerides, a type of healthy fat.

Substitutes:
- Use maple syrup instead of honey.

Tips:
- Roll the bites in extra matcha powder for a vibrant look.

Turmeric Golden Milk Popsicles

Preparation Time: 15 minutes (plus freezing time)
Yield: 6 popsicles
Caloric Count: Approximately 70 calories per popsicle

Ingredients:
- 2 cups coconut milk
- 1 teaspoon turmeric powder
- 1/2 teaspoon ground cinnamon
- 1/4 teaspoon ginger powder
- 2 tablespoons honey
- A pinch of black pepper

Method of Preparation:
1. In a blender, mix coconut milk, turmeric powder, cinnamon, ginger powder, honey, and black pepper.
2. Empty the mixture into popsicle molds and freeze until solid.

Health Benefits:
- Turmeric has anti-inflammatory properties that may help with menopausal symptoms.

- Coconut milk offers healthy fats for hormonal balance.

Substitutes:
- Use almond milk instead of coconut milk.

Tips:
Incorporate a few slices of fresh ginger for an extra kick.

Protein-Packed Greek Yogurt Parfait

Preparation Time: 10 minutes
Yield: 2 servings
Caloric Count: Approximately 160 calories per serving

Ingredients:
- 1 cup Greek yogurt
- 1/2 cup granola (preferably low-sugar)
- 1/2 cup mixed berries (strawberries, blueberries)
- 1 tablespoon honey

Method of Preparation:
1. In a glass, add in layers, the Greek yogurt, granola, and mixed berries.
2. Repeat the layers.
3. Drizzle with honey before serving.

Health Benefits:
- Greek yogurt provides probiotics for gut health.
- Berries offer antioxidants that support overall well-being.

Substitutes:
Opt for maple syrup instead of honey.

Tips:
- For added fiber, add a sprinkle of chia seeds

Sweet Potato and Cinnamon Muffins

Preparation Time: 30 minutes
Yield: 8 muffins
Caloric Count: Approximately 120 calories per muffin

Ingredients:
- 1 cup mashed sweet potato
- 1/4 cup coconut flour
- 1/4 cup almond flour
- 1/4 cup honey
- 2 eggs
- 1 teaspoon cinnamon
- 1/2 teaspoon baking soda
- A pinch of salt

Method of Preparation:
1. Preheat oven to 350°F (175°C) and line a muffin tin with paper liners.
2. In a bowl, mix mashed sweet potato, coconut flour, almond flour, honey, eggs, cinnamon, baking soda, and salt.
3. Divide the batter into muffin cups and bake for 20-22 minutes.

Health Benefits:
- Sweet potatoes provide beta-carotene, essential for skin health.
- Cinnamon may have anti-inflammatory effects.

Substitutes:
-Opt for maple syrup instead of honey.

Tips:
- For added creaminess, top with a dollop of Greek yogurt.

Mango and Coconut Chia Popsicles

Preparation Time: 15 minutes (plus freezing time)
Yield: 6 popsicles
Caloric Count: Approximately 90 calories per popsicle

Ingredients:
- 1 cup mango, diced
- 1 cup coconut milk
- 2 tablespoons chia seeds
- 1 tablespoon honey
- 1 teaspoon lime juice

Method of Preparation:
1. In a blender, puree mango, coconut milk, chia seeds, honey, and lime juice.
2. Empty the mixture into popsicle molds and freeze until solid.

Health Benefits:
- Mangoes are rich in vitamins A and C, supporting immune health.
- Chia seeds are highly abundant in omega-3 fatty acids and fiber.

Substitutes:
- Use almond milk instead of coconut milk.

Tips:
- Add some mint leaves for a refreshing twist.

Baked Apple with Cinnamon and Walnuts

Preparation Time: 30 minutes
Yield: 2 servings

Caloric Count: Approximately 130 calories per serving

Ingredients:
- 2 apples, cored and halved
- 2 tablespoons chopped walnuts
- 1 tablespoon honey
- 1 teaspoon cinnamon
- A pinch of nutmeg

Method of Preparation:
1. Preheat oven to 375°F (190°C).
2. Place apple halves in a baking dish.
3. In a bowl, mix chopped walnuts, honey, cinnamon, and nutmeg.
4. Fill each apple half with the walnut mixture.
5. Bake for 20-25 minutes until apples are tender.

Health Benefits:
- Apples are rich in fiber, supporting digestive health.
- Walnuts provide omega-3 fatty acids, beneficial for heart health.

Substitutes:
- Use maple syrup instead of honey.

Tips:
-For added creaminess, top with a dollop of Greek yogurt

CHAPTER THIRTEEN

BEVERAGES, HERBAL TEAS AND SMOOTHIES

Mango Tango Smoothie

Preparation Time: 10 minutes
Yield: 2 servings
Caloric Count: Approximately 150 calories per serving

Ingredients:
1 cup frozen mango chunks
1/2 cup Greek yogurt
1/2 cup almond milk
1 tablespoon chia seeds
1 teaspoon honey
Ice cubes (optional)

Method of Preparation:
In a blender, combine frozen mango chunks, Greek yogurt, almond milk, chia seeds, and honey.
Blend until smooth.
Add ice cubes if desired and blend again.

Health Benefits:
Mangoes contain vitamins A and C, supporting immune health.
Chia seeds are highly abundant in omega-3 fatty acids and fiber.
Substitutes:
Use coconut milk instead of almond milk.

Tips:
Garnish with a slice of fresh mango for a decorative touch.
 Berry Bliss Smoothie Bowl
Preparation Time: 15 minutes
Yield: 2 servings
Caloric Count: Approximately 180 calories per serving

Ingredients:
1 cup mixed berries (strawberries, blueberries, raspberries)
1/2 banana, sliced
1/2 cup spinach leaves
1/2 cup almond milk
2 tablespoons Greek yogurt
1 tablespoon almond butter
Granola and sliced almonds for topping

Method of Preparation:
In a blender, blend mixed berries, banana, spinach leaves, almond milk, Greek yogurt, and almond butter until smooth.
Pour into bowls and top with granola and sliced almonds.

Health Benefits:
Berries are rich in antioxidants that may reduce inflammation.
Spinach provides iron, important for energy production.

Substitutes:
Use peanut butter instead of almond butter.

Tips:
Customize with additional toppings like chia seeds or shredded coconut.

Green Goddess Detox Smoothie

Preparation Time: 12 minutes
Yield: 2 servings
Caloric Count: Approximately 120 calories per serving

Ingredients:
1 cup kale, stems removed

1/2 cucumber, peeled and sliced
1/2 green apple, cored and chopped
1/2 lemon, juiced
1 tablespoon fresh ginger, grated
1 cup coconut water
Ice cubes (optional)

Method of Preparation:
In a blender, combine kale, cucumber, green
apple, lemon juice, ginger, and coconut water.
Blend until smooth.
Add ice cubes if desired and blend again.

Health Benefits:
Kale is rich in calcium and vitamin K,
supporting bone health.
Cucumber provides hydration and is low in
calories.

Substitutes:
Use spinach instead of kale.

Tips:
Sip slowly to savor the refreshing taste.

Turmeric Spice Golden Milk

Preparation Time: 15 minutes
Yield: 2 servings
Caloric Count: Approximately 80 calories per serving

Ingredients:
2 cups almond milk
1 teaspoon turmeric powder
1/2 teaspoon cinnamon
1/4 teaspoon ginger powder
1 tablespoon honey
A pinch of black pepper

Method of Preparation:
In a non stick saucepan, heat almond milk over medium heat.
Add turmeric powder, cinnamon, ginger powder, honey, and black pepper.
Whisk until well combined and heated through.

Health Benefits:
Turmeric has anti-inflammatory properties that may help with menopausal symptoms.
Almond milk provides vitamin E, essential for skin health.

Substitutes:
Use coconut milk instead of almond milk.

Tips:
Enjoy before bedtime for a relaxing treat.

Coconut Berry Hydration Elixir

Preparation Time: 10 minutes
Yield: 2 servings
Caloric Count: Approximately 100 calories per serving

Ingredients:
1 cup coconut water
1/2 cup mixed berries (strawberries, blueberries, raspberries)
1 tablespoon fresh mint leaves, chopped
1 tablespoon chia seeds
1/2 lime, juiced
Ice cubes (optional)

Method of Preparation:
In a blender, blend coconut water, mixed berries, mint leaves, chia seeds, and lime juice until well combined.
Pour over ice if desired.

Health Benefits:
Coconut water is hydrating and contains electrolytes.
Berries provide vitamins and antioxidants.

Substitutes:
Use basil leaves instead of mint.

Tips:
Adjust sweetness with a drizzle of honey if needed.

Pineapple Ginger Zing Smoothie

Preparation Time: 12 minutes
Yield: 2 servings
Caloric Count: Approximately 140 calories per serving

Ingredients:
1 cup pineapple chunks
1/2 banana
1/2 teaspoon fresh ginger, grated
1 cup coconut water
1 tablespoon flaxseeds
Ice cubes (optional)

Method of Preparation:
In a blender, blend pineapple chunks, banana, ginger, coconut water, and flaxseeds until smooth.
Add ice cubes if desired and blend again.

Health Benefits:
Pineapples contain an enzyme called bromelain, which reduces inflammation.
Ginger may help alleviate nausea and support digestion.

Substitutes:
Use mango instead of pineapple.

Tips:
Add a fresh pineapple slice as a garnish to add a touch of the tropics.

Beetroot Berry Power Smoothie

Preparation Time: 15 minutes
Yield: 2 servings
Caloric Count: Approximately 160 calories per serving

Ingredients:
1 small beetroot, peeled and chopped
1/2 cup mixed berries (strawberries, blueberries)
1/2 cup Greek yogurt
1 tablespoon chia seeds
1 tablespoon honey
1 cup water
Ice cubes (optional)

Method of Preparation:
In a blender, blend beetroot, mixed berries, Greek yogurt, chia seeds, honey, and water until smooth.
Add ice cubes if desired and blend again.

Health Benefits:
Nitrates found in beetroots may improve athletic performance.
Greek yogurt provides probiotics for gut health.
Substitutes:
Use almond milk instead of water.

Tips:
Adjust sweetness with more honey if desired.

Cinnamon Apple Pie Smoothie

Preparation Time: 12 minutes
Yield: 2 servings
Caloric Count: Approximately 130 calories per serving

Ingredients:
1 apple, cored and chopped
1/2 banana
1 cup almond milk
1/2 teaspoon cinnamon
1 tablespoon almond butter
1 tablespoon ground flaxseeds

Ice cubes (optional)

Method of Preparation:
In a blender, blend apple, banana, almond milk, cinnamon, almond butter, and flaxseeds until smooth.
Add ice cubes if desired and blend again.

Health Benefits:
Apples provide fiber, aiding in digestive health.
Cinnamon may help regulate blood sugar levels.
Substitutes:
Use peanut butter instead of almond butter.

Tips:
Add a sprinkling of cinnamon on top for garnish.

Matcha Mint Refresher

Preparation Time: 10 minutes
Yield: 2 servings
Caloric Count: Approximately 90 calories per serving

Ingredients:
1 teaspoon matcha green tea powder
1 cup almond milk
1 tablespoon fresh mint leaves, chopped

1/2 teaspoon honey
1/2 teaspoon vanilla extract
Ice cubes (optional)

Method of Preparation:
In a glass, whisk matcha powder with a small amount of almond milk to create a paste.
Add the rest of the almond milk, mint leaves, honey, and vanilla extract. Stir well.
Pour over ice if desired.

Health Benefits:
Matcha green tea provides antioxidants and may enhance mental alertness.
Mint may aid in digestion and soothe nausea.

Substitutes:
Use coconut milk instead of almond milk.

Tips:
Sip mindfully to savor the refreshing taste.

Orange Creamsicle Smoothie

Preparation Time: 12 minutes
Yield: 2 servings
Caloric Count: Approximately 120 calories per serving

Ingredients:
1 cup orange segments
1/2 banana
1/2 cup Greek yogurt
1/2 teaspoon vanilla extract
1 tablespoon chia seeds
Ice cubes (optional)

Method of Preparation:
In a blender, blend orange segments, banana, Greek yogurt, vanilla extract, and chia seeds until smooth.
Add ice cubes if desired and blend again.

Health Benefits:
Oranges are high in vitamin C, supporting immune health.
Greek yogurt provides protein for satiety.

Substitutes:
Use honey instead of chia seeds for sweetness.

Tips:
Garnish with a slice of orange for visual appeal.

Cranberry Citrus Antioxidant Infusion

Preparation Time: 15 minutes
Yield: 2 servings
Caloric Count: Approximately 100 calories per serving

Ingredients:
1/2 cup cranberries (fresh or frozen)
1 orange, peeled and segmented
1/2 lemon, sliced
1 tablespoon honey
1 tablespoon fresh mint leaves, chopped
4 cups water

Method of Preparation:
In a pitcher, combine cranberries, orange segments, lemon slices, honey, and mint leaves.
Add water and stir well.
Let it chill in the refrigerator for at least 2 hours before serving.

Health Benefits:
Cranberries are rich in antioxidants that may promote urinary tract health.
Citrus fruits provide vitamin C, essential for collagen production.

Substitutes:
Use lime instead of lemon for a different citrus flavor.

Tips:
Serve over ice for a refreshing experience.

Blueberry Basil Brain Boost Smoothie

Preparation Time: 12 minutes
Yield: 2 servings
Caloric Count: Approximately 110 calories per serving

Ingredients:
1 cup blueberries (fresh or frozen)
1/2 cup basil leaves
1/2 banana
1 cup almond milk
1 tablespoon flaxseeds
Ice cubes (optional)

Method of Preparation:
In a blender, blend blueberries, basil leaves, banana, almond milk, and flaxseeds until smooth.
Add ice cubes if desired and blend again.

Health Benefits:
Blueberries contain antioxidants that may support brain health.
Basil may have anti-inflammatory and adaptogenic properties.

Substitutes:
Use coconut water instead of almond milk.

Tips:
Enjoy as a mid-morning or afternoon pick-me-up.

Peaches and Cream Protein Smoothie

Preparation Time: 12 minutes
Yield: 2 servings
Caloric Count: Approximately 130 calories per serving

Ingredients:
1 cup sliced peaches (fresh or frozen)
1/2 cup Greek yogurt
1/2 cup almond milk
1/2 teaspoon vanilla extract
1 scoop vanilla protein powder
Ice cubes (optional)

Method of Preparation:
In a blender, blend sliced peaches, Greek yogurt, almond milk, vanilla extract, and protein powder until smooth.
Add ice cubes if desired and blend again.

Health Benefits:
Peaches provide vitamins A and C, contributing to skin health.
Greek yogurt offers protein for muscle maintenance.

Substitutes:
Use honey for added sweetness.

Tips:
Choose a high-quality protein powder for optimal nutritional benefits.

Minty Watermelon Quencher

Preparation Time: 10 minutes
Yield: 2 servings
Caloric Count: Approximately 90 calories per serving

Ingredients:
2 cups watermelon, diced
1 tablespoon fresh mint leaves, chopped
1 tablespoon lime juice

1/2 teaspoon honey
2 cups coconut water
Ice cubes (optional)

Method of Preparation:
In a blender, blend watermelon, mint leaves, lime juice, and honey until smooth.
Pour into glasses and add coconut water.
Stir well and add ice cubes if desired.

Health Benefits:
Watermelon is hydrating and contains vitamins A and C.
Mint may aid in digestion and provide a refreshing taste.

Substitutes:
Use basil leaves instead of mint.

Tips:
Serve in a chilled glass for a cooling effect.

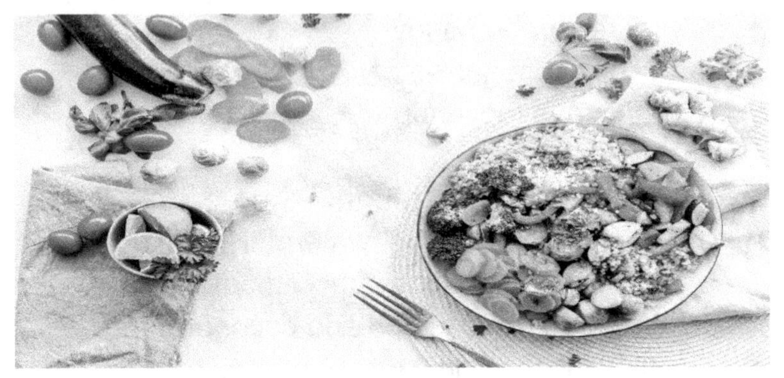

APPENDIX

Your Daily Planner

Studies indicate that those who maintain a daily log of their food intake have significantly greater success in maintaining their health and reducing their weight compared to those who do not. Keep a journal of the recipes you attempt during your eating window while on intermittent fasting and the physical changes that occur in your body with this daily planner. This will not only give you an excellent summary of your development, but it will also serve as a useful guide for you going forward as you pursue your health goals.

DAYS	RECIPES	REMARKS

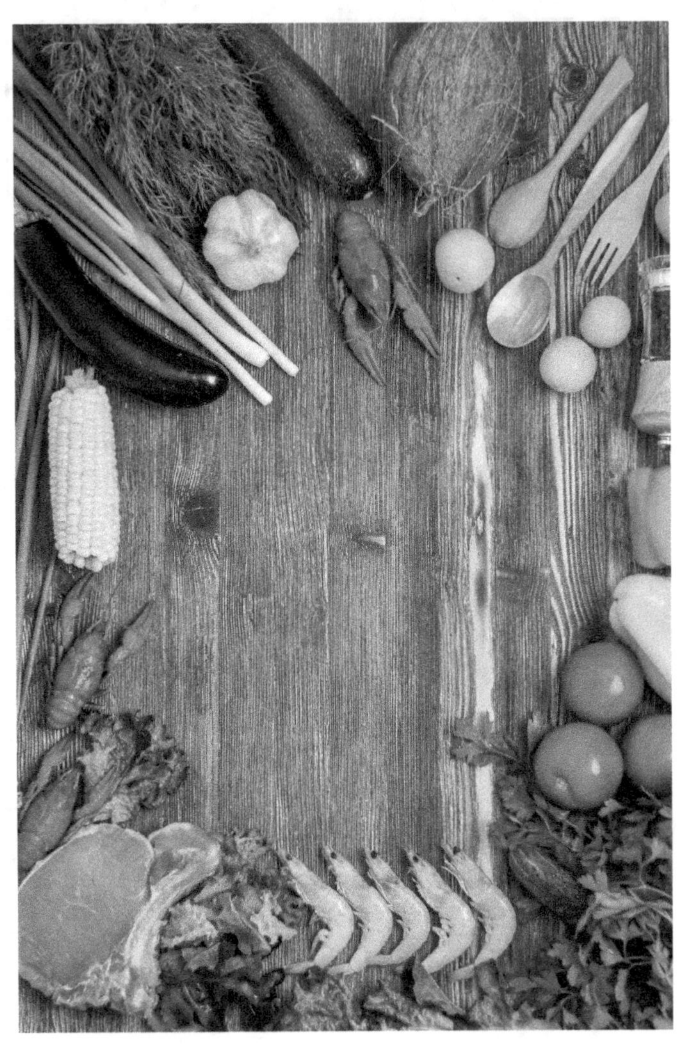

CONCLUSION

In conclusion, intermittent fasting has emerged as a popular and effective weight loss and health improvement strategy, particularly for women over 50. By incorporating intermittent fasting into your daily routine, you can enjoy numerous benefits, such as improved overall health, increased longevity, and a reduced risk of chronic diseases. Moreover, you can enjoy the flexibility of eating your favorite foods without feeling restricted or deprived, making it a sustainable and enjoyable approach to healthy living.

As you embark on your journey with intermittent fasting, remember to:

- Consult with a healthcare professional to ensure that fasting is appropriate for your individual needs and health conditions.
- Monitor your progress and adjust your fasting routine as needed to optimize its benefits.
- Stay committed to your fasting schedule and maintain a balanced diet to achieve your health goals.

By following these guidelines and embracing the principles of intermittent fasting, you can unlock the potential for a healthier, more vibrant life. Remember, the key to success lies in consistency and finding a fasting routine that works best for you and your lifestyle. Happy fasting!

REVIEW O' CLOCK

HOW DID WE DO?

Have you experimented with the recipes in our Intermittent Fasting for women over 50? Did our recipes make managing your health easier and more delicious? We'd love to hear your thoughts. Please share your feedback with us. This is how we improve.

Positive reviews and insights from wonderful customers like you, will help others feel confident about choosing this book and can guide those who are looking for a helpful resource to manage their health-related issues through healthy cooking.

Thank You and Happy Cooking!

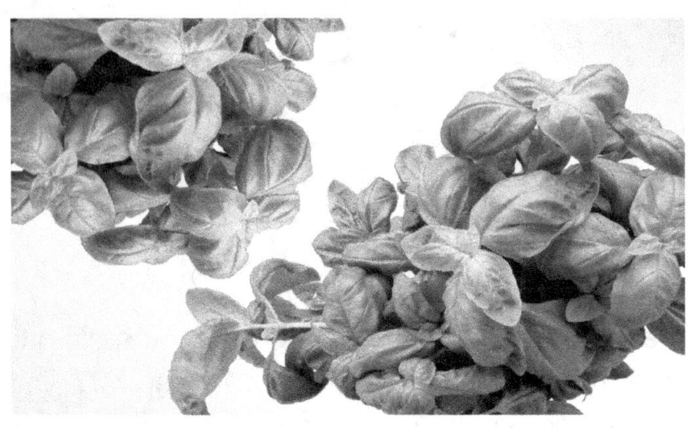